ISBN: 9798393115210

Love a Wholistic Life, Inc.

Cover and original illustrations, Kate Brand

Headshot photography, Zac Poor

DEDICATION

DEDICATION

This book is dedicated to my dad Jerry Hill.
Daddy, you have the heart of a lion. Strong and
fierce. Your journey has given Beth and I purpose.
Your love and wisdom have given us direction.
We could not have done this without you!

Thank you for your love and commitment.
Thank you for choosing us to be your daughters.

"In case after case, Christen Kaplan works miracles for my clients who must lose massive amounts of weight before they can undergo surgery from accident and injury, in some cases, eliminating the need for surgery altogether." *Charlie Perez, CEO, Medical Acquisition Company, Inc.*

"I was asked to lose weight and be in the best shape possible prior to spinal surgery. Christen's unique communication skills allowed me to transition to heightened physical and mental well-being. It wasn't a diet, it was lifestyle change that I have continued to maintain years later." *Thomas Hilt*

"I just love Christen! I could never have done this without her. She knows what she is talking about. I lost 47 pounds, and my doctor was happy to decrease my diabetes medications because I did not need them anymore. It was a journey but definitely worth it!" *Sheryl Faver*

"[Kaplan's] program is powerful! I lost 40 pounds and am no longer pre-diabetic. My blood pressure is down and I feel amazing. Thank you, Christen! Best coach ever!" *Jesus Sian*

"I had all the signs of a troubled digestive tract, resulting in a fatty liver. My liver panel went back to normal in six weeks after starting on Christen's plan. I'm staying on the program for life." *K. Larcomb*

TURN YOUR HEART AROUND!

Book 1 in

Christen Kaplan's

TAKE BACK YOUR HEALTH!

Series

CONTENTS

TURN YOUR HEART AROUND!

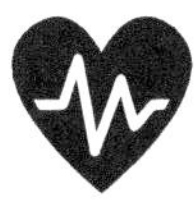

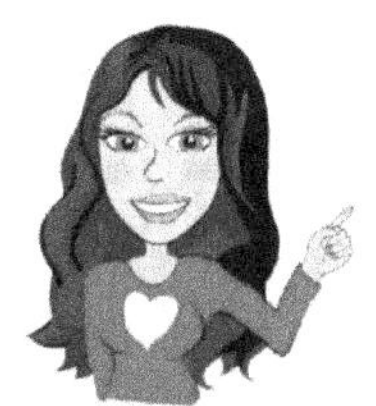

HOLD IT! STOP RIGHT THERE! *Christen here, and I see you! Don't be like me and skip this introduction, because there's some really important information in here, and I don't want you to miss it.*

With nearly 75% of Americans overweight and in the obese categories, and as a result, unable to maintain basic health, it's highly likely you (or someone close to you) is facing a life-threatening health challenge right now. No matter where you are in your life journey, no matter how impossible your current mental, physical, emotional, and spiritual state seems to be, with courage, perseverance, and willingness to focus your energy in a new direction, you can put yourself on the path to take back your health. I know this to be true because my family did it, and I did it too!

This powerful book represents a radical departure from much of what you find in the self-help and nutrition community. I am not a doctor. I am not a therapist. I am a Certified Holistic Nutritionist and Wellness Expert with over 20 years' experience helping people just like you reclaim their health. But, this book isn't all about nutrition. This book addresses specific lifestyle diseases such as heart disease, high cholesterol, high blood pressure, and type-2 diabetes, illustrated by personal accounts of how my father fought through lifestyle disease, and won the battle.

In America, the number one cause of death is heart disease. Most heart diseases are considered preventable lifestyle diseases. An overwhelming body of medical research from authorities such as Harvard Medical Journal, Cleveland Medical Clinic, the Center for Disease Control (CDC), World Health Organization (WHO), and many other credible re-sources agree that over 80% of chronic diseases affecting Americans today are driven by lifestyle factors such as diet and exercise.

This book, *Turn Your Heart Around - The Mind, Body, & Soul Connection to Prevent and Reverse Lifestyle Disease*, explains in easy-to-understand terms what lifestyle diseases are and how you can overcome them to take back your health.

You will learn how these diseases have taken America by storm and how to avoid and reverse the damage these life-threatening diseases have caused.

I will share my dad's challenging journey to reclaim his health, along with my own personal confrontation with poor health, and the emotional roadblocks that threw me off course along the way. I do this because I want you to know I get it. I have been where you are, and I'm here to tell you, you can turn your heart and your health around. My hope is that on some level, you will identify with our stories and make use of the tools I developed over twenty years as a wellness and nutrition expert, helping people fight their way back to great health.

Your journey won't be easy. Change doesn't happen overnight. But I can assure you, if you are willing to confront those obstacles that have been holding you back, clean your mental house, and use the tools presented in this series, you will find your way to a happier, healthier you.

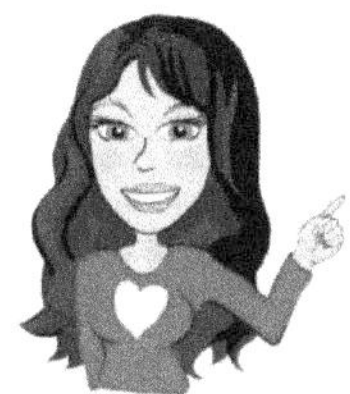

FAIR WARNING: *Some of the material I share in this series will be raw and uncensored. It's important for you to know the truth, not a glossed-over version of it.*

I'm passionate about this work, and my style is no-holds-barred. I fight every day for my clients' lives and I will fight for yours if you stay the course.

We'll start with the first steps of my dad's journey and some sobering facts. I'll share some of my own experiences, so let's not waste time; let's get to work.

In Search of a Treasure

Think of your journey as the treasure map of your life, and you are the creator. Open your mind to embrace the new ideas. In this book you will find all the tools you need to take control of your own health. I will offer you the nutritional advice that has literally turned my clients' lives around. Many who had one foot in the grave have regained not only their physical health, but are also living happy and peaceful lives, full of gratitude for the many unexpected treasures they discovered along the way.

As a Certified Holistic Nutritionist and Health and Wellness Expert, I help people create the quality of life they have always wanted by teaching them how to own the outcome of a healthy and abundant life. My life so far has been a crazy journey that has led to happiness, peace, health, and gratitude. It has gifted me compassion and understanding which helps me guide my clients to a place of self-love and acceptance. I help them build courage to take a leap of faith and believe in themselves. With compassion and under-standing, I lead them until it is safe to let them walk alone. Eventually that walk becomes a happy skip to a fulfilling, healthy life.

I am sure many of you have experienced some pretty messed up "BS" in your life. Please know you are safe here. I come from a place of no judgment what-soever. You will see as you read further that I get it. I understand you. I went through some crazy crap too.

My own journey led me to where I am today, and I choose to live with no regrets. I would do it all over again to be where I am today. People say that all the time, but do they mean it? I can say I do. Because with all the BS comes an opportunity to learn major life lessons that will serve you well in the future, even if it doesn't feel like an opportunity at the time. Just wait because those lessons are coming.

There will be some laughter and some tears while reading this book. You will celebrate some victories and face some hard life choices. However, when you reach the end of this book, I can assure you, you will not be the same person you were when you started.

Working through this process can bring some things to the surface that could be difficult to handle. You may come to the realization that you need some additional support. There is no shame in asking for help. There are amazing professionals out there qualified to help if you're struggling with deep issues you can't navigate on your own. I am a big believer that maintaining your mental health is just as important as maintaining your physical health. Your mental health is housed in your body so that should only make sense.

IMPORTANT: This book is not intended as a substitute for professional mental health care.

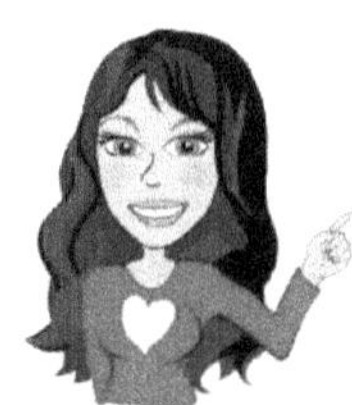

I like to check in with my therapist when I am overwhelmed and need someone to help me help myself. She is a Godsend when I need help self-correcting.

If you do not already have a relationship with a mental health care provider, check the back of this book for resources that may be helpful.

NOTES

Please take advantage of these notes pages to write down your thoughts as you work through this book.

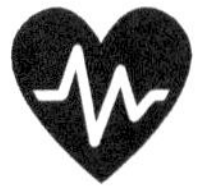

I sat on the plane staring out the window into the emptiness of the sky, my head spinning, as tears ran down my face. My heart was sinking deeply. Desperation and anxiety overcame me at the thought of my father unconscious and helpless as he lay on the surgical table. Just two hours before my flight I had received an urgent phone call that my father had been rushed into the operating room for emergency open heart surgery.

The doctors told my family there was a 95% chance he would not come off the surgical table alive. You see, my father weighed almost 600 pounds and his heart was giving out. He had type-2 diabetes, cardiovascular disease, peripheral artery disease, loss of kidney function (due to his diabetes), high cholesterol, and extremely high blood pressure. All I could do was pray that I would get there in time to say goodbye.

The most heartbreaking thing about that day was that every medical condition that put him on that table facing what could be his last breath was considered a Lifestyle Disease.

What is Lifestyle Disease?

Oxford Language describes Lifestyle Disease as: Any medical disorder or condition thought to be produced or exacerbated by aspects of a person's lifestyle choices such as diet, day-to-day habits, and physical inactivity, all chronic behaviors that make it impossible to maintain basic health.

Let's look at some important statistics:

- Heart Disease is the number one killer in the United States of both men and women.

- As of this writing, the CDC says 74.6% of Americans are overweight or obese. (30.7% overweight, and 42.4% obese.)

- These numbers are going up 5% a year.

- 1 out of 10 Americans is morbidly obese, that is, they have serious health conditions that can interfere with their basic physical functions such as breathing or walking.

- 70% of all adults use at least one prescription medication a day; 70% of adults 40 to 75 years old use up to five or more prescription meds a day.

- 70% of adults in the United States use prescription drugs for mental health.

- The top 5 drugs sold in the United States are prescribed for high blood pressure, diabetes, high cholesterol, anti-stress and anxiety, and anti-depression.

What Does it Mean?

So, what does this all mean for you and me? It means lifestyle disease affects our overall wellbeing and not just the state of our physical bodies. There is so much more to being healthy. To reach optimum health, we need to reach a state of homeostasis or balance within our physical, emotional, and mental health as well as our social wellbeing.

It means there is a connection between your physical body and its needs, as well as your emotional and spiritual needs. To support a healthy life, you must be able to thrive mentally, physically, and socially. It means that you must tap into your own personal courage to take back your health. Are you starting to see the pattern?

Health and courage go hand-in-hand. You are going to hear these terms over and over, so let's take a look at the definitions:

The World Health Organization defines *health* as: A state of complete physical, mental, and social wellbeing and not merely the absence of disease.

Oxford Languages defines the word *courage* as: Strength in the face of pain or grief.

Webster's Dictionary defines *courage* as: Mental or moral strength to resist opposition, danger, or hardship, and firmness of mind or will in the face of extreme difficulties.

Extreme Situations

The most common thread I see in the people who come to me for help is they have all experienced at one time or other, usually when they were very young, an extreme situation that caused serious damage to their spirit.

Extreme situations can influence your journey. Maybe you were in an accident, or maybe someone in your life was excessively hurtful and abusive when you were a child.

What's important to understand as we start this journey together is that you choose how you respond to these people or circumstances. You choose whether you will give your power away or use it to learn and grow through those hurtful situations. Everyone, and I mean everyone, has had experiences in their lives that paralyzed them emotionally or mentally at one time or another. As children, that experience is when we first realize there is something wrong in the world, or something wrong with ourselves.

There is a saying I love from iconic motivational speaker, Zig Ziglar: "There will always be people in your life who treat you wrong. Be sure to thank them for making you strong!"

I know I have a lot of people to thank and I'm guessing you do, too.

Peacefulness vs Happiness

How do you define happiness? For me, happiness is more of an emotion, while peacefulness is a state of mind, that is, being in a state of peacefulness. My happiness is being at peace with my choices and in my relationships with the people I love.

Many people believe they will not find happiness until everything in their life is perfect. That is a huge, impossible expectation. In a perfect world, we would all be the perfect height and weight, with the perfect education, job, house, wife, husband, and children, driving the perfect car. In that world, we would have nothing by which to gauge a happy life. That's why perfection is impossible, and your journey is so important.

Happiness comes in so many ways. We all have individual ideas about what makes us happy, but nothing will make you happy until you realize the most important factor in being happy: Happiness comes when you can accept and love yourself.

I am 54 years old. I am in a place in my life where things do not have to be perfect. Problems are not problems to me, they are challenges, a chance to learn, problem solve, and conquer. The ability to look at challenges that way means I have something to gain out of the experience. You may be thinking to yourself "does she mean every problem?"

Yes, I mean every problem.

When I reflect on my 54 years and all the devastating and emotionally crippling experiences I've gone through, I can truly find a lesson learned in every one of those circumstances. I may not have seen them at the time, but now the lessons are so clear. Since I adopted this mindset years ago, I live a much more peaceful life full of happiness because when a problem arises, I look at it as an opportunity to problem solve and learn an important life lesson.

The journey to take back your health will be bumpy and seem impossible at times but hold on tight. There is hope. Whether you've gotten the first news from your doctor that something must change, or your health has been spiraling out of control for a long time, the tools I am going to give you can pull you back from the edge and put you on the path to better health.

Just to be clear: I am not a doctor. I am not a therapist. I am a Certified Holistic Nutritionist and Wellness Expert. I have had my own battles with my health and weight in the past. I know what it feels like to be unhealthy, and I also know what it feels like to be healthy! Most importantly, I have walked the walk with nutrition, and I know for a fact, hands down, that you can change your life, health, and body through good nutrition.

We have a lot to share and learn together, so, let's keep going and see where your journey will take you.

First Steps

Before you read any further, grab yourself a pen and keep it handy. Be ready to write down your thoughts in the Journal and Notes pages throughout this book. Write all over this book for that matter. (If you're reading this on an eReader, get yourself a notebook and keep it handy as you go.) That is what this book is for. Read it, ponder the message, use it as a workbook to apply it to your individual circumstance.

Peeling back the layers of the emotional, spiritual, and physical elements of your experiences and writing them down for future use will help you start your personal journey with your eyes wide open and embrace the world of possibilities within your unique potential.

NOTES

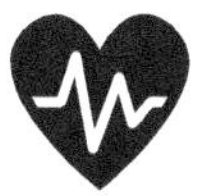

I arrived at the hospital in time to participate in the family frantically trying to figure out what steps would come next in preparation for my father's funeral. We needed to figure out who would handle what and how we would share in helping my mother adjust to life without her husband of almost 40 years. I felt like I had stepped out of my body and was watching a drama on TV. I was a daddy's girl. My dad walked on water as far as I was concerned. He was the Patriarch of our family, our pillar of strength. He was the one I bombarded with all my dilemmas, and he always had the right answers for me. He was my hero. I simply couldn't process what my life would be like without my dad.

After what seemed like forever, the surgeon finally walked through the double doors to the hospital waiting room with an exhausted look on his face. I fully expected to hear the words "I am sorry but… "

Instead, he looked at my mom, smiled, and said "I do not know how he did it Mrs. Hill, but your husband made it through the surgery. He is in recovery and will be transferred to the Intensive Care Unit for close observation. I hope he appreciates the miracle that just happened. Your husband flatlined during the procedure but clearly his will to live was stronger than his willingness to die. He should recover but he will have to make several major lifestyle changes, or he won't be this lucky the next time. You can see him in about an hour. The nurse will come and get you."

We were overcome with emotion as you could imagine and all I could think of was that God clearly was not ready for my dad yet, and my dad clearly was not ready to die.

My mom went in to see him first. Twenty minutes later she came back to the waiting room and looked straight at me. "Sissy, daddy wants to see you… alone."

I pushed myself out of the chair my butt had been glued to for hours, my heart pounding fiercely in my chest. I had prayed for the chance to have one more conversation with my dad, and thank God, and by some miracle, I was now going to get it. You see, at that time I was a Certified Nutritionist, a Medical Exercise Specialist, and Post Rehab Specialist. I prayed that God would use me to help my dad someday, but most importantly that my dad would accept my help.

It was still pretty dark as I walked into the ICU Unit, but the light from the hall outside was enough to let me see his tear-filled eyes. Before I could say anything, he said, "Sissy, I do not want to die."

My heart broke for him. This was the first time I had ever seen my dad cry and be so vulnerable.

I gently hugged him and kissed his forehead. "Daddy, God gave you a second chance. If you want to live, you have to change your eating habits and some of your lifestyle choices. Do you think you can do that?"

To my relief, he softly whispered, "Yes."

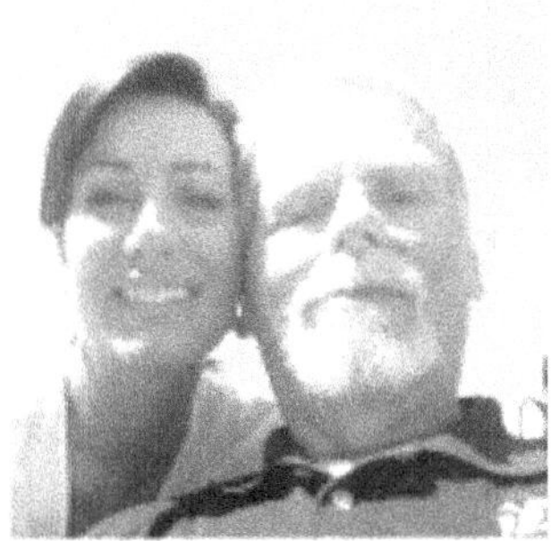

Dad and me

We continued to chat for a little while longer. I promised him I would move home for the next four months to help him through what would become his journey to take back his health.

But his is not the only story. With the large majority of people in the United States suffering from lifestyle-related disease, it's likely someone in your family, or a close friend, is facing the same reality. My oldest brother suffered from heart disease, extremely high blood pressure, gastro-esophageal reflux disease, type-2 diabetes, high-cholesterol, and kidney failure (walking in my father's footsteps).

My youngest brother is currently suffering from gout, gastroesophageal reflux disease, extremely high blood pressure, and high cholesterol. My mom suffered from type-2 diabetes, high blood pressure, high cholesterol, gastroesophageal reflux disease, breast cancer, and complications due to drug interactions from taking multiple prescription medications. My grandfather died in his mid-fifties due to lung cancer. He was a smoker. My family is not much different than most American families. The only difference is that this family has two Certified Holistic Nutrition-ists in it (me and my sister) and we are going to keep fighting for our family and yours!

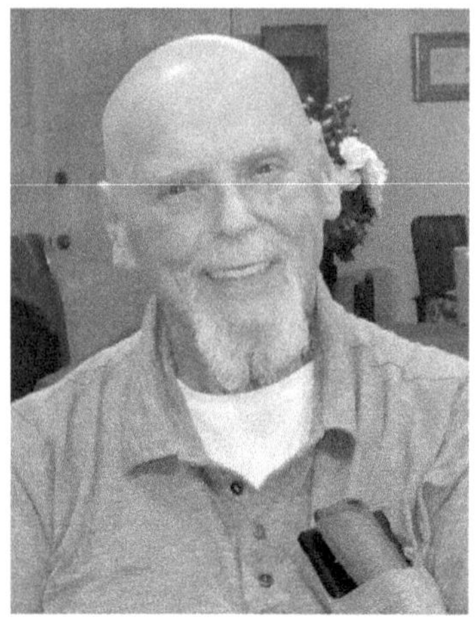

Dad after losing 375 pounds

My dad's story is just one of millions every day about people in remarkably simi-lar circumstances. How-ever, unlike most, his story has a happy ending.

He went on to lose 375 pounds. It took him a year and a half, but he was able to get off most of the med-ications he was on.

He is no longer a type-2 diabetic, and God gifted him several more years to spend with his family and his grandchildren.

He worked hard… extremely hard. There were lots of tears, many colorful words, and a few arguments, but I'm relieved to say, he never gave up. Thirteen years later, my dad is 76 years old, and he isn't going anywhere soon, God willing.

He is my hero! He overcame an extreme situation to take back his life and his journey. He fought like hell and pulled his own foot out of the grave. He did it… He did all the work and was relentless until he reached his goal. He should not be alive today, but he is because he took control of his journey, and his journey was far from over.

If my dad could overcome and take back his health against what seemed like impossible obstacles and make major lifestyle changes, there is truly hope for everyone, which means: There is hope for you.

A Piece of Me

I am going to share more of my personal journey with you throughout this book. It is not pretty at times, so I want you to be aware, some material in this book series will be intense, raw, and uncensored. I will share not only my story, but stories of others close to me whose journey got really freaking hard before it got much easier. Some stories may be alarming or frightening, but they are also stories of major breakthroughs and redemption.

You will probably see some of yourself in these stories and some of this will land pretty hard on you. But remember, it takes courage to see what is in front of you.

Remember When You Were Young

When we are young, we are fearless. We take our health for granted. We eat whatever we want, and for many of us our metabolism burns through it with no problem. (When I was in my twenties my go-to food was pizza, basically every day, along with a two-liter bottle of Mountain Dew.)

As a young person you wake up every day full of energy. You can even pull all-nighters and function the next day like you got a blissful eight hours of sleep. You can party like a rock star and not suffer a hangover. Life is good when you are young.

The thirties are not so bad. You are still in the prime of your life, but life becomes real, and you start taking on the stressors of adult responsibilities such as marriage, kids, paying off student loans, buying a home, paying bills, and trying to get ahead in your career.

Maybe you're not married but looking for your person. The search for Mr. or Miss right, especially in today's online dating culture, can create a plethora of confusion and stress. Unfortunately, this I also know from experience. (I could, and probably will write a book on that topic. It would be a true comedy, but let's not digress.) My point is, life is changing, and by your thirties, the stress load is starting to pile up on you.

Then you hit forty and things change again. In addition to the stresses of your thirties, now you're starting to put on a little weight, you're not making it to the gym because you are way too busy. Your eating habits are still the same as when you were young, but your metabolism is not, and your body is suffering. You're not sleeping as well, and it starts to show. Your job is stressing you out. Trying to keep up with family, relationships, and financial responsibilities starts to weigh you down.

You go to your doctor and he or she says you need to drop a few pounds, you are prediabetic, your blood pressure is getting a little high, and you need to keep your eye on your cholesterol. They will most likely give you some prescription medications to help you manage these symptoms. Oh, and while we're at it, let's throw in some prescription meds to help you manage your stress.

Sound familiar? If it does, this is a major red flag. This is your body screaming at you for help! This is your body telling you it can't hold out for long before it quits on you. This is your body begging you to love it and fix it so it can continue to support you and provide for you.

It's time to gather your courage and say it with me: "Take Back Your Health!"

How We Got Here

Let's backtrack even more and start at the beginning. Your journey began the moment your mama labored, and your little head came popping out of her… let's just say womb. You took your first breath and then communicated to everyone in the delivery room that you were not happy with your bright, new environment. You wanted your mommy.

That was the beginning of learning to communicate your feelings and you caught on fast. You learned if you cry, mommy or daddy will come running to put you at ease. If you are hungry, you cry. If your diaper needs changing, you cry. If you are tired and need a nap, you cry. Your parents learned very quickly how to comfort their little precious one.

As you get a little older and are learning how to use your words to communicate, your parents start asking you what you need. Are you hungry? Do you need to go potty? Do you want to play with your toys? Do you want mommy to read you a book? Important choices when you're a toddler.

When you become an adolescent, however, your choices start to have consequences. If your mom says stay out of the cookies and you get into the cookie jar and eat them anyway, you get yourself in trouble. You start to learn that maybe that was not the best choice. It's funny when you think about it; there is a reason God makes babies so cute. Your parents do not have to teach you how to misbehave, they spend a lot of their parenting time teaching you how to behave.

Our natural instincts when we are young are self-serving. When my youngest daughter was little, she used to take toys out of her friends' hands when she wanted to play with them. Her friends would cry and I had to teach her that it wasn't nice and that it hurt her friend's feelings when she did that. She had a very precious heart when she was a toddler (thankfully still does). It wasn't long before she was picking up toys to proudly hand to her friends to make them feel better.

Your teen years become a whirlwind of good and poor choices as the learning curve prepares you for adulthood. Keep in mind, your brain is still developing, and hormones are raging throughout your teenage body. As teens, we often internalize the mistakes we make, and sometimes they tend to become part of our identity. They can be deeply embedded roadblocks to our healthy development. We haven't had enough life experience to know these are learning experiences meant to teach us how to problem solve.

If you are a parent to a teenage daughter who tends to be hyper-emotional, you can clearly relate to this. In general, most girls go through a crazy roller coaster ride of emotions throughout their teen years and boy do they love to talk. This is because of the large amount of the female hormone, estrogen flooding their body. If I ask my teen daughter how her day was, I anticipate a lengthy description of her day. If I ask my teenage son how his day was, I am lucky to get a shrug or maybe a three-word answer such as "it was okay." Boys have a completely different experience through their teen years than girls do. They have a huge amount of the male hormone, testosterone surging through their body. They just want to be left alone, to be fed, and they often become very competitive, and this is normal behavior for a teen boy.

Whether you are a boy or girl, your teen years are critical for your development, physically, mentally, and emotionally.

Your Parents' Job

Your parents' job is to safely release you into society at age 18, hopefully, as a good human being ready to contribute to society, armed with a strong moral compass and values that will guide your future choices. In other words, you are now well into your own personal journey. Your parents are no longer legally responsible for your choices. It becomes very clear when you are a young adult there is an outcome to every choice you make. Here comes the tough part. As a young adult you do not have the life experience of knowing up front if some of your choices are the right ones. It is easy to be influenced by friends.

According to the National Institute of Health, a young person's brain is not fully developed until the age of 25. The University of Rochester Medical Center says that it doesn't matter how smart teens are, the rational part of a teen's brain isn't developed until the age of 25, when the prefrontal cortex is finally fully developed. This is why parents become confused when their extremely intelligent kid seems at times to lack common sense.

As you can see, your journey starts way before you realize you're in control of your own choices. These choices have either positive outcomes or negative consequences. Let's peel back another layer of this epiphany. The first time you realized there was something wrong with the world or wrong with yourself is when you had a shift in your development from the innocence of a child living in their imagination, to beginning to experience fear and uncertainty. You begin to experience feelings you have never felt before and that can be scary. This is where we start developing roadblocks in our personal journeys.

My Precious Little One

It is funny, as a mom to a teenage girl, I can see where my daughter is going to trip and fall through her teenage years. I try to advise her and hope she doesn't trip but I know she will need to for certain life lessons to resonate with her to help her to make some better life choices in her future.

I can only protect her from so much because she must go on her own life journey. It is painful to think about, sometimes very painful. I can pick her up and brush her off, pat her on her ass and send her out again but that is all I can do. Her dad and I are simply her coaches. She is the captain of her own team. She must catch what we throw at her and run with it. Sometimes, she makes a touchdown and sometimes she gets crushed by the opposition. I am sure you can relate, especially if you are a parent.

The point is, even as children, we are all responsible for our own journey. My mama-bear instincts want to control her every move, but if I want her to thrive and not just survive in this world, I have to let her make her own choices and be responsible for the outcome.

Embrace Your Journey

I have no way to know what stage of your journey you are currently in, whether you're just starting out, or facing some frightening, difficult circumstances because of a lifetime of poor lifestyle choices. However, I want you to learn to embrace your own journey and ride the wave in and out, understanding that every step is a precious learning experience that leads you to where you are supposed to be. Your journey does not end at a pot of gold at the end of the rainbow as most people would like to think.

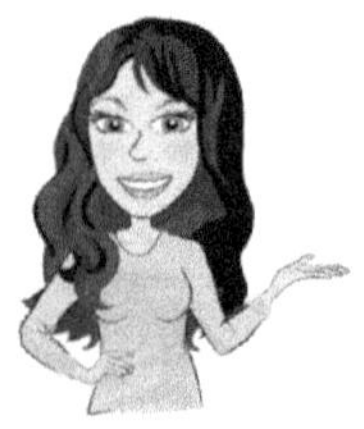

Where you think your journey is going is never where you end up. I promise it will be better than that. Grasp the wisdom and understand that your journey belongs to only you.

You hold the power behind each choice you make. The bad news is that once you realize this, you must take responsibility for where you currently are in your life. You may have to own and clean up a few messes. The great news is, with responsibility comes the freedom to create whatever you desire for your life. You have the freedom to make whatever choice you want to move forward in your journey.

Once you understand the importance of embracing your own journey, everything begins to make sense. The "Ah Ha" moments start to pour in, and you can finally enjoy the process of achieving your wants and desires without fear. You will feel empowered to soldier through the necessary steps to reclaim your desired health which leads to your desired life. This sounds like a pipe dream, right? I promise you, it is not. It is entirely possible when you discover the courage to love yourself and make it so, mind, body, and spirit.

At this point you might be beating yourself up a little for not taking responsibility for your own journey sooner. Please go easy on yourself. What I've learned over the last twenty years is that people simply don't know what they don't know. And that's okay. This book is about a journey of discovery. I'm here to help you fill in some of those blanks and set you on a solid footing to take back your health.

Making it Personal

It's time to find a quiet place where you can take a few moments to reflect on what you've read. I want you to think about responsibilities in your life that may feel overwhelming right now. Write them all down. (Remember this is a "no judge" zone.) Maybe it's parenting challenges, or simply getting out of bed in the morning. I will ask you to return to these later in your journey when we begin *Chapter 6 – Meditation/Prayer* and learn how to turn perceived problems into challenges and challenges into life lessons.

JOURNAL

TURN YOUR HEART AROUND

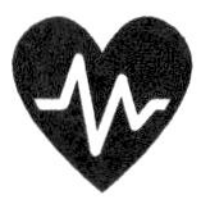

Twenty years ago, I was sitting at a restaurant with my boyfriend and noticed with alarm that everywhere I looked were overweight people. My heart started to race in my chest. I leaned over and whispered to him, "We need to leave… *now*."

He was a little taken aback by my attitude but agreed without resistance. When we got in the car, I immediately started complaining about all the big people in the restaurant. I was so angry at them; all of them. My boyfriend was surprised at my reaction to these people; people I didn't even know. Like most men, he didn't react. He just drove quietly and let me rage. It didn't take long for me to realize he was not going to engage or support anything I had to say. I sat in the car during the ride home, sick to my stomach, fiercely internalizing my harsh, judgmental attitude.

Until then I had never considered myself to be a judgmental person, but for some reason in that moment, my emotions exploded inside me. Why had I attached such strong feelings to these innocent people just trying to enjoy a meal with their friends and loved ones?

When I got home, I called a good friend who happened to be a family therapist. I explained to him my ridiculous outburst and my internal upset directed at the patrons of the restaurant. He asked me to come in at the end of the week and I agreed.

I had not seen my friend, Jim as a therapist nor had I seen any therapist for that matter. Back then only broken people went to see therapists. At least that's what I thought growing up. Mental healthcare was not something people talked about back then. I have to admit though, to have had such harsh feelings toward strangers I do not know meant I had something inside of me that needed to be fixed and I was praying Jim would help me fix it.

I arrived at his office 15 minutes early, extremely nervous but ready to spill my guts. I hoped he had some answers for me other than I was just being a judgmental bitch. When he called me into his office, he could see I was truly upset. We started talking about what happened at the restaurant, then he moved on to questions about my family.

"Is anyone in your family overweight?"

"My father and oldest brother are both morbidly obese," I said.

"What was a normal meal like at your house?"

I was about to give him whatever details I could think of, and then my heart squeezed tight as a vivid memory grabbed me, a scene I hadn't thought about until he asked. "Before we were excused, us kids used to pass our plates of unfinished food down the table to my dad and he would eat whatever was left on our plates." There were six of us, so he was consuming a great deal of extra food.

"So, Christen," he asked, "Are you angry at your father or brother for being overweight?"

Really? What kind of question was that? "Of course not!" I countered.

But he persisted. "Are you sure?"

My heart sank and then I looked down and said "No, I am not sure."

I was in the first year of my training as a Certified Personal Trainer and I had just become certified as a nutritionist.

"And why do you think you chose to become a CPT and a nutritionist?"

The lightbulb went on, and the truth hit me upside the head: At that time, my dad was over 500 pounds, and my brother was over 400 pounds. I was subconsciously angry at my dad and my brother for being so morbidly obese. I felt so ashamed for being angry at my dad and my brother whom I loved so much, I shifted my angry reaction to other obese people because I had been unable to tell my dad or brother how I felt.

The next thirty minutes were a blur. I vomited my anger and upset all over Jim. He just sat there and listened while I cried and raged on. As my session came to an end, he reminded me that I had positioned myself in my career to help people like my dad. People who are sick and morbidly obese need someone who can relate to their battle with their health and weight. He suggested I could find redemption in serving other people who really need my help.

I went back to my car and sat in the driver's seat. As I looked into the rear-view mirror at the image of my face: snotty nose, mascara everywhere, puffy blood-shot eyes. It became very clear in that moment that my calling was to love, support, and help those who simply do not know what they do not know. I know for a fact that neither my dad nor my brother had any idea things would go horribly wrong for them because of the food they were eating, until it was too late.

Uncovering Deep Seeded Fear

I discovered I had held unresolved anger toward my family members for placing me in a state of fear for their lives. It was a very humbling turning point in my life. A revelation. I wasn't angry at the people in the restaurant, I was living in fear that my father's eating habits were going to kill him and that my brother was following in his footsteps. Fear can be paralyzing and manifest in unexpected ways in all areas of your life.

I cannot speak for the dynamics in your family, I can only speak for mine. It is very painful watching a loved one self-destruct because of eating the wrong foods. Here's what I learned. If you are in an unhealthy situation due to excessive weight gain, the threat to your life deeply affects *everyone* in your family. You say, "It is my body, why should anyone else care?" The answer to that is, your family loves you and they, like me, do not want to lose you prematurely. You are needed and valued even if you do not think so right now.

I worried about Dad from the time I was very young until he finally made the choice to get healthy. He was "gifted" his life back and he did not waste that gift. He was not ready to say goodbye to his wife and family. Often, we do not love and value ourselves the way our family loves and values us. I remember many times as a young adult, thinking every time the phone rang and it would be my mother about to tell me something had happened to my dad. Fear would strike my heart almost every time she called.

In my thirties I dreaded asking my parents how they were doing because I could see my dad was getting bigger and bigger and my mother became obese as well.

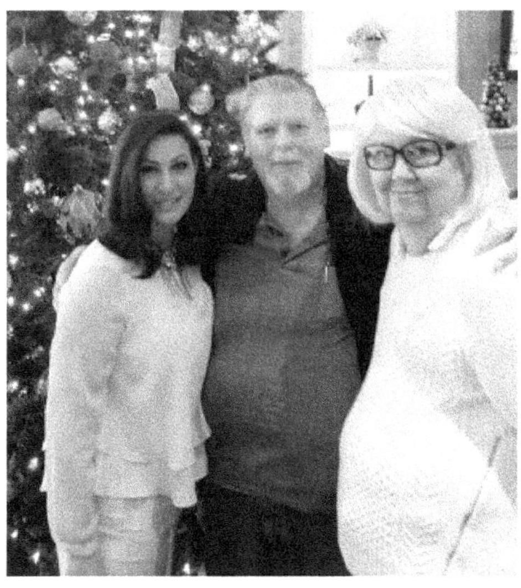

Mom, Dad, and me

It was painfully obvious their health was spiraling out of control. Neither of my parents could walk across the room without breaking a sweat.

Dad's diabetes was restricting circulation to his lower legs, and they were turning purple.

His kidney's started taking a hit and he lost significant kidney function, all due to diabetes. Food had a hold of my dad, and it wasn't letting go.

My mom became addicted to food and progressed to diabetic as well. If she got a wound on her foot or leg, it took forever for the wound to heal because there was no circulation in her lower legs and feet. It broke my heart.

Knowledge is Power

Knowledge is power my friends. I can't emphasize that enough. My parents, like most people, had no idea the foods they were putting in their bodies were killing them.

My dad faced certain death on that operating table and was gifted a second chance. When he started feeding his body nutrient-rich foods and feeling the difference, the light came on in his brain: This profound change in his eating habits was saving his life. Eating healing foods became a "No Brainer" for him. From now on he will choose healthy foods over facing certain death. (Okay, he might enjoy a slice of pizza now and then, but he *knows* where falling back into old habits will take him and he's not going there ever again.)

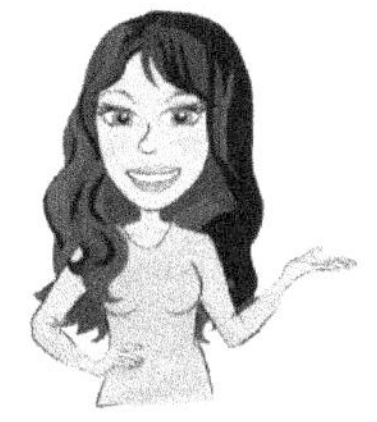

Now that my father has lost the excess weight and has taken back his health, you cannot get the man to sit down. He will tell you that he has too much life to live to sit around.

The Standard American Diet (SAD)

Let's take a moment to consider what you don't know about food.

Oxford languages defines food as: Any <u>nutritious</u> substance that people or animals eat or drink or that plants absorb in order to <u>maintain life and growth</u>.

Encyclopedia Britannica describes food as: A substance consisting essentially of protein, carbohydrates, fat, and other <u>nutrients</u> used in the body of an organism to <u>sustain growth and vital processes</u> and to <u>furnish energy</u>.

Dictionary. Com's definition of food: Any nourishing substance that is eaten or consumed or otherwise taken into the body to sustain life and provide growth and energy.

Does the Standard American Diet fit these definitions of food? No, it does not, which is why I'll be referring to it from here on as the SAD diet. The SAD diet not only lacks any nutritional value, but it is also killing people instead of maintaining life. I would not call the SAD diet actual food. It is just an edible substance. That's it. In fact, except for the *growth* part, the SAD diet does the opposite, (but I am quite confident the definitions weren't referring to obesity as growth.)

Real food contains the nutrients the body needs to thrive and maintain life. Your food should not be your worst enemy. Unfortunately, the SAD diet is exactly that.

Let's continue to uncover and understand what you may not know about yourself that may be keeping you from taking back your health.

When the Tables Turn

Let's talk about getting "judgy" for a moment and think about how that feels. As I shared in the beginning of this chapter, deep seeded fears about losing my father made me bristle with anger when I saw overweight people in a restaurant. I didn't know this about myself until I got to the bottom of it, recognized it for what it was, and learned to let all that go.

Karma kicked me in the ass; let me tell you what happened when I was at my heaviest.

I was in my car with my daughter in a grocery store parking lot when a man nearly t-boned us. No one got hurt, but the thought of my daughter coming that close to being hurt in an accident scared me to death. When I honked at him, he purposely blocked my car so I could not move. I hopped out, and marched over to the driver, ready to give him a piece of my mind.

He rolled down his window and before I could say a word, he yelled at me: "You fat *effing* bitch!" Then he hit the gas and drove away.

He certainly deserved a tongue lashing for nearly causing an accident, but those hateful words stopped me in my tracks. My self-image had taken a beating since I'd put on a lot of weight. I forgot all about my anger as those words sunk deep. They stuck with me for weeks. This time I was the one being judged, and it hurt.

These are the kinds of things we hold on to that we do not know are lurking below the surface, ready to sabotage us.

Making it Personal

Okay, it's time to visit your quiet place again, get out your pen, and think about a time when you were judged by someone you didn't even know, or maybe it was someone close to you and it cut you to the bone, and still bothers you today. Use the following Journal pages to write it down.

JOURNAL

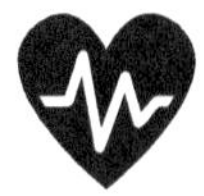

We're going to confront fear head on in this chapter, so hold on to your hat. Hopefully as we move throughout this book you will be able to identify the areas in your life where fear has paralyzed you or become a subconscious form of self-sabotaging and self-defeating behavior in your journey up to this point.

What things do you think of when you think of fear? What are you afraid of?

Here's my list in no specific order:

- I am afraid of anything happening to my family or my friends that would remove them from my life or cause them pain. Examples would be an accident, sickness, and God forbid, death.

- I am afraid of scary movies. I hate scary movies. My sister LOVES them! I still haven't figured that out! If you met her, you would never guess that one!

- I am afraid of big spiders... Yuck!!!! A big spider would send me running for the hills screaming like a little girl!

- I am afraid of tidal waves. I used to have nightmares about them but not anymore.

- I am afraid of losing my purpose and not being able to help people in my career.

- I am afraid of my sister dying before me. She is my soulmate. I cannot imagine my life without her.

- I am afraid of losing any of my children.

- I am afraid of losing my health and living in pain and suffering with no quality of life.

- I am afraid of a zombie apocalypse, just kidding, although you never know.

- I used to be afraid of rejection. Did the work on myself so that is no longer a fear.

- I used to be afraid of dreaming big. I worked hard on that one. Now there are no limits to what I can do, and I thrive on that energy.

- I used to be afraid of not being accepted or not being good enough. Again, did the work on myself so I am no longer afraid of that.

- I used to be afraid I would never find love again after divorce. Again, did the work on myself and am now confident and trust the process. I enjoy being single, but I have become open to the right man being a part of my life when the time and person are right.

Do you get the point? There are many forms of fear. If you look at my list, most of the things I'm afraid of things that are out of my control and attached to things that I have made up. I most certainly cannot control tidal waves, spiders, someone I love getting sick, or even when it's their time to leave this world. Yet these things still strike fear in my heart when I think about them. However, the logical and rational side of me knows these things are 100% out of my control. So, I choose not to allow the things I cannot control to strike fear in me. Let's take a closer look at how fear manifests in our lives and how we can take control.

Things You Can't Control

There are things you can control and things you cannot. I used to be afraid of being rejected by my now ex-husband.

When we were going through challenges in our marriage, I acted out of that fear often and that made things worse, not better.

After a while, I grew to realize that my behavior hurt me a lot more than it hurt him. I also realized that wanting to hurt someone because they hurt me was also a response to fear. I was so worried about keeping score with my ex-husband for the things he had done to hurt me in our marriage, I started acting and reacting in a way that only fueled the fire and made things worse. I eventually recognized that acting out of fear was a self-defeating behavior that was turning me into someone I did not internally want to be; someone I didn't recognize.

I had to do a lot of work on myself after my divorce to find forgiveness, compassion, and to soften my heart so I could put my family back together again.

My ex and I worked very hard to build trust in our relationship and become a family again. Each of us was responsible for the destruction of our marriage and we both knew it. After a lot of humbling therapy, we have built a strong family unit for ourselves and most importantly for our children.

Divorce does not have to destroy families. There does not have to be a bad guy when the marriage ends. We are a stronger family unit now than when we were married. We started focusing on cleaning up on our own side of the street and focused on forgiveness instead of keeping score. We stopped reacting out of fear.

We began to look for ways to support each other as parents and as friends.

It was not easy. I had to keep reminding myself that I was not responsible for the choices my ex made. I had to leave his garbage on his side of the street and get back to cleaning my side. I learned the biggest lessons in my life going through that clean-up process. If you do not clean up your own mess, no matter how justified you feel in making it, you will never evolve into the better, wiser version of yourself.

I also confronted a lot of fears I was unaware I was subconsciously harboring. I learned to become the person I was proud of and stop blaming my ex and others for my unhappiness. He was not responsible for my choices, and I most certainly was not responsible for his. I stopped suffering the consequences of his choices and stopped trying to make him suffer the consequences of mine.

Nothing feels better than owning your mess and cleaning it up. There is freedom in growing through those life lessons. Pay attention to your responses during times of conflict. Are you reacting out of fear? What are you afraid of? One of the most profound things my therapist shared with me is that when you are yelling or screaming at someone, you are reacting out of fear. You can't clean that up unless you recognize what is really going on there.

He also told me it is an emotionally abusive act to lose the ability to control your anger and yell and scream at your spouse (or anyone else for that matter).

That landed hard on me because I grew up with parents who never yelled at each other, ever. To this day I have never heard either my mom or my dad say even one hurtful word to each other. My marriage was not so lucky.

It took a few years, some therapy, and a lot of self-reflection and hard work but things could not have turned out better. My ex is now my friend, and I am blessed to have him as the father of my children. He is a good man and an excellent father because *we* worked hard, and because *I* raised him up instead of continuing to knock him down. The outcome is so much better when you raise someone up because in that scenario, everyone wins.

There is a saying, "If you look for the worst in someone you will find it. If you look for the best in someone you will find it." That is definitely something you *can* control.

I want to touch on one last thing on this subject. I took a three-day seminar by Alison Armstrong called *Understanding Men*. One thing she says in her seminar is that men, in general, will rise to the occasion if you just lift the men in your life up. I lift my ex-husband up with praise and thank yous for being a great father, and for every other positive thing he does. Almost every time I do, he exceeds my expectations.

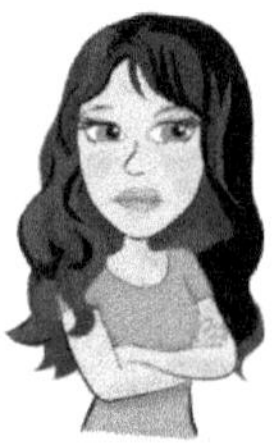

IMPORTANT: *Not every situation merits staying the course in a relationship. In the event you are in an abusive situation your fear is justified and you may have to remove yourself completely from the relationship and seek professional help.*

If you need help with an abusive or frightening situation and do not know where to turn, be sure to check in the Resources section in the back of the book for information that may help you address these issues.

Things You Can Control

For years I gave over my control to people who did not have my best interests at heart. I allowed myself to become emotionally paralyzed by fear of rejection, fear of losing my purpose, fear of not being good enough. It took time and a lot of work on myself to learn that I held the power and control over my journey, and that no one could take that away from me unless I willingly let them.

Confronting fear takes courage. (There's that word again.) To become courageous, you must first see who you really are. When you strip back the layers of fear, you can acknowledge the power that you may have allowed others to have over you. Let's look at an example of how that can happen.

When I was a little girl my best friend Kim and I used to go to the playground and pretend we were prima-ballerinas. We made tutus out of anything we could wrap around our waists and our grass-stained tennis shoes made excellent ballet slippers. We were six years old, and we were convinced that one day we would be super famous ballerinas. When we leaped into the air it truly felt like we were at least six feet off the ground. Were we six feet off the ground? No… maybe six inches, but when you are a little girl your imagination is your reality. I believed I was flying through the air with grace and precision.

One day after Saturday morning cartoons, Kim and I raced to the playground to practice our ballet moves. Two teenage girls were there smoking cigarettes by the slide. Kim and I didn't care, we continued playing and dancing all over the playground. After about ten minutes flying high in our imaginations, the girls called us over. I was convinced that they were in awe of our dance skills and that they were going to tell us how amazing we were. We skipped over to them ready to absorb all the rave reviews that we were sure they were going to shower on us. One of the girls, who seemed to be the alpha of the two, had long stringy blond hair and was wearing what I assume was her boyfriend's high school jacket, a popular thing to do back then. It symbolized you were taken and evidently made you special. I do not remember much about the other girl other than she had short dark hair and wore bright pink lipstick.

As we arrived in front of the girls, I noticed they were not smiling. As a matter of fact, they scowled at us and informed us this was "their turf" and we needed to get our "mother-*effing*" asses off their playground. Kim froze, but without even thinking, I shouted back at them "No!" then went on to inform stringy-blonde-haired-girl we were famous ballerinas, and this was *our* dance studio!

The next thing I knew the blonde girl smacked me in the mouth and pushed me down onto the asphalt. I was stunned. I couldn't feel anything but pain shooting up my tailbone. She then glared at me and said "You will never be a famous ballerina! You jump around like a frog, and you are as ugly as a frog!" Then they walked away laughing.

I can remember that moment so clearly because that was the first time I realized there was something wrong in the world and it was the first time I realized there was something wrong with me.

I left my dream of being a famous ballerina on the playground that day and would never leap through the air again. I handed my power over to two teenage girls that I didn't even know. Two girls that I am sure never thought of me again or lost one second of sleep over that brief exchange.

For years I believed the horrible things miss Stringy-Blonde-Haired Girl said to me. I believed I was as ugly as a frog. I believed I would never become a famous ballerina. I stopped dancing. I stopped dreaming and imagining. In that moment, I started seeing the world differently. Why would someone do that to me? When you first realize there is something wrong in the world or something wrong with you it stunts your ability to live blissfully as a young child in your imagination. It can emotionally paralyze you as it did me for a long time.

After the girls left, Kim helped me up. She was so proud of how I stood up to the older girls.

I refused to let her see me cry so I fought back the tears and listened to her praise my bravery as we walked back to my house. When I arrived home, I went to the bathroom and washed the dirt and blood off my face. My lip was swollen, and my tailbone was sore. I went to my bedroom, laid down in my bed, and silently wept until I fell asleep. I never told my parents what happened. When my father asked me what happened to my lip I lied and told him I fell off the monkey bars. Which, by the way, was the beginning of me learning to cover up my hurt.

Unresolved conflict or circumstances can paralyze us for years. Because I had no resolution to the playground conflict, the inner turmoil and pain it created stayed with me for years. As difficult as it is going to be, you have to go back and identify those circumstances. I'm not going to lie, it's going to be painful, but you can resolve the actual circumstances. The way to do that is to be your own superhero. Imagine you are your own superhero right now. What would you say to that younger you to help resolve that conflict?

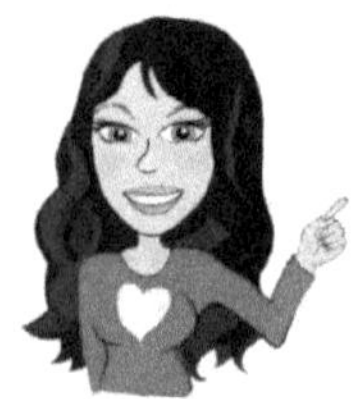

Obviously, when you're six, you can't internalize or assess the emotional damage done by being assaulted and having your dreams torn to shreds. That day on the playground set in motion the transfer of a precious power that only little innocent ones possess. I let Stringy-Blonde-Haired Girl rob me of my dreams and the imagination so critical to a child's development.

Whether you are a child, or an adult who has suffered abuse of any kind at the hands of someone else, it is not only hurtful, it can also be devastating and cause lasting trauma that will follow you throughout your life if you do not eventually confront those "demons" and take back your power.

Recognizing Vulnerability

You do not have to be a child to give your power over to someone else. All of us at some time or another have surrendered our power to someone else, especially when we are going through a crisis or a particularly devastating time. In this mental state, we are particularly susceptible to fear.

It's important to recognize that when we're in a particularly vulnerable situation in our lives, some people will take advantage. Fear of rejection and loss of security can sometime cause us to turn our power over to someone else because we don't feel strong enough to make it on our own.

But know this, there is no shame in recognizing vulnerability, or that you have given your power over to someone else. Some of us feel guilty that we made a bad choice during a vulnerable time. If that is you, you need to go easy on yourself.

We have this misconception that every mistake we've ever made makes us a bad person; that mistakes can somehow outweigh the goodness in us. We start to identify ourselves by the mistakes we've made instead of the lesson we learned from those mistakes.

If you knew going in you would learn a great lesson from a possible mistake, you wouldn't be afraid to forge ahead with something that could turn out to be a great learning experience.

Think of the expectations we put on ourselves when everything has to be perfect! That level of expectation is exhausting and impossible to maintain. If every time you make a mistake, you kick yourself, you forget to retrieve the lesson.

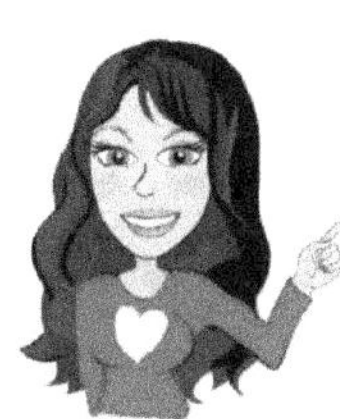

REMEMBER: *Mistakes do not define you; they are meant to help you learn. Learn to recognize when you are vulnerable and guard against those who would take advantage.*

All of us have experienced rejection at some point in our lives. Fear of rejection can be extremely painful to work through. I have a friend, let's call her Ashley, who is a very loving, kind, and generous person. She has the most precious heart, and I love her to death. She is one of the funniest people I have ever met. I absolutely cherish her. Unfortunately, she allows other people into her life who do not have the best intentions. As smart as she is, I am often not only surprised but baffled by some of her choices. One day we had a long discussion over coffee, and she poured her guts out to me about a relationship she was in and was fighting to hold on to.

Every area of her life is solid. She is very talented, has a great job, she is fun to be around, and she is beautiful. You would think she held the world in her hands. However, she was in a relationship with someone who did not treat her with love and respect. He cheated on her, lied to her, yelled at her, and called her names. I was completely horrified to hear she was suffering in such a dysfunctional relationship. I believed she could have the pick of the litter. She had everything going for her and was the full package. Why would she fight for a relationship with someone who did not value her? As she went on, I had a "Dr. Phil" moment, and I had to stop her and ask her an important question.

"Ashley, when you were a little girl did you have a lot of friends?"

"Yes, why?" she replied.

"Can we go off topic for a moment? What was it like growing up with your friends?" I sat back and listened to her reply, surprised at her answer.

She shared with me a lot of fun times at first, but then she clutched her hands in her lap and shared a very painful situation that made a lot of sense once she explained it. Her childhood friend, let's call her Natalie, was her best friend from the age of three. They were inseparable. Natalie meant everything to her. When Ashley was twelve, Natalie transferred to another school and Ashley stayed behind at the school they had both attended most of their young lives. They stayed in contact but spent less and less time together as time went by. The following year Ashley transferred to the same school her best friend was attending.

Ashley was so excited to be back with her bestie and was over the top with joy to be sharing classes with her again. She was convinced everything was going to go back to normal and that she and Natalie would take Jr. High by storm together.

When the first day of school came, she naturally assumed Natalie would introduce her to her group of friends. It would be so much easier to blend in with new friends having her BFF by her side. But her actual experience wasn't easy at all. It was a disaster.

When she arrived at school, she waited for Natalie by the lockers. She saw Natalie and some of her friends walking down the hall coming toward her. Excitement grew inside her as she practiced in her head all the things she would say to her best friend and new friend group. To her astonishment and deep pain, they walked right past her and did not acknowledge Ashley at all. Ashley was devastated. She ran behind them and caught up with Natalie.

She pulled on Natalie's arm and said, "Hey, I was waiting for you by the lockers."

Her best friend barely acknowledged her and kept walking.

It was the deepest heartbreak Ashley had ever felt. She ran to the bathroom and cried.

The relationship between Ashley and Natalie dissolved and eventually Ashley found another friend group. This time Ashley made sure she was seen and heard in her friend group. Unfortunately, this group of friends were not a good influence on Ashley. She ended up making some very poor choices.

Her grades went from straight A's to flunking. Her parents were shocked and brokenhearted as they witnessed the changes in their daughter. Luckily, it did not take long to identify why Ashley was suffering so much at the school she was attending. Eventually, Ashley's parents had no other choice but to transfer her to a new school so she could have a fresh start. Ashley's life turned around and she started to thrive again. However, one thing became obvious to her after becoming an adult. Fear of rejection was still deep seeded in Ashley.

I am sure as you are reading this now you can think of someone in your life you held on to even though they mistreated you. Fear of rejection can take control of you and cause a plethora of problems and disfunction in your life. Fear of rejection can leave a path of destruction and destroy your confidence and self-worth.

It was heart breaking to see my good friend struggle through this messy relationship.

As we sat in the café that day, I advised Ashley to speak with someone who could help her work through that painful experience. At first, she was reluctant, but eventually she broke down and started seeing a therapist. Within a few months, Ashley ended the relationship with the man she was once obsessed with. She now recognizes that fear of rejection had a tight grip on her, keeping her in a relationship that was unhealthy and difunctional.

Could this be you? Take some inventory. Are you a people pleaser because you are afraid you will be rejected?

Do you stay in relationships with friends, romantic interests, coworkers, or even family members who do not value you because you fear being rejected?

You are not alone. We are tribal creatures by instinct. The group of people we have around us are our tribe. We all have a natural instinct and desire to be part of a group. Your tribe provides structure and security and the thought of being banned from that "tribe" can be devastating. It took many life lessons and "break-ups" for me to finally learn that I have the power to choose my tribe, my tribe does not choose me. I protect myself and my family by surrounding myself with people who I know have my back and love me fiercely. I, in turn, offer the same love and support to them. You have the right and power to choose who you want in your tribe so choose your tribe wisely.

Recognizing Fear in Others

It is important to understand that when people hurt you, or are emotionally or physically abusive to you, it is an expression of *their own* fear and their own insecurities. Abuse is not normal or acceptable behavior. Something is terribly wrong in the abuser's life or their journey that is creating that mess. I can only imagine what teenage Stringy-Blonde-Haired-Girl's home life must have been like for her to be so angry she would strike a little six-year-old girl. Being first rejected and then assaulted by Stringy-Blond-Haired-Girl tore away at my innocence and left me wounded for years.

You can't control other people's choices or behaviors, but you can control your choices and response to their behavior. You can choose to willingly hand over your power, or you can take back your power and do what is right for you and your journey. You should never live in misery to make someone else happy.

If I could go back to my six-year-old self, I would pick that precious little girl up and wrap her in my arms. I would share so many things with her. I would tell her that she is beautiful, that she is incredibly talented and that she is going to grow up and become a successful powerhouse of a woman. I would tell her to not to be afraid. I would kiss her forehead and tell her she is so smart and that she is going to go on an amazing journey that is full of twists and turns that will challenge her but thrill her at the same time.

I would tell her she can and will create an incredible life for herself serving others and helping them live fulfilling and healthy lives. I would tell her she was personally touched by God when she was born, that she is deeply loved, and that she in turn will love deeply and make a difference in people's lives. Then I would love on her some more and send her off on her journey armed once again with the confidence, imagination, and creativity that was stripped from her.

It is possible to let go of childhood trauma and find redemption. I know because I did it by being my own Superhero.

Making it Personal

Think about the areas in your life where fear of a person or a circumstance has emotionally paralyzed you.

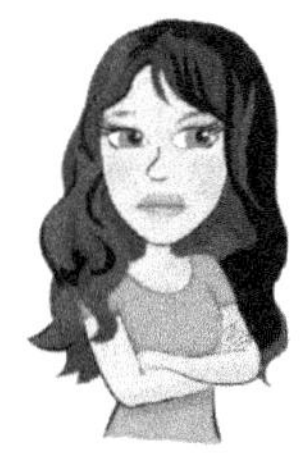

REMEMBER: *Fear can be your worst enemy. It can strip you of your freedom and drain your power. It's time to have an honest conversation with yourself about times in your life when you gave away your power.*

Do you use these people or circumstances as an excuse to not take responsibility for where you are in your life? No one is going to judge your answers.

This is a chance to show love and respect to yourself by being honest and owning those choices.

Once you can identify these critical moments and choices, you can begin the healing process as I did when I got real with myself.

All right. It's time to put that pen to work. Use the following journal space to write down your thoughts. I'm going to give you lots of space here, because facing our fears is a huge part of removing the roadblocks to making meaningful lifestyle changes.

Make a list of the things you have been afraid of,
then ask yourself: Are these fears rational?
Which ones do I have control over? Which ones are
out of my control?

Did you give your power away to someone by
making them responsible for your fear?
Did you surrender your control when you were
feeling vulnerable?

If you could go back in time as your own superhero,
how would you help that child through their
trauma? How would you love that child?

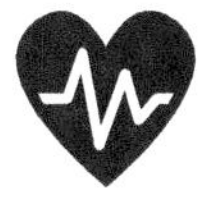

I started my first business when I was 27 years old. I was living in Chicago at the time. Obsessed with fashion and make-up, I had been modeling from a young age and when I wasn't in front of a camera, I was behind it doing make-up for photoshoots and fashion shows. It was a crazy but fun time in my life, as your twenties often are. I had arrived back in Chicago from a trip I took to Miami's South Beach where I had been working on a fashion show. One of the things I was known for as a makeup artist was my ability to constantly mix colors to get exactly the right shade of foundation and lip color I had envisioned for the model or for the fashion designer's vision.

At the end of the show, as I was cleaning and packing up my station, one of the lead hair stylists approached me and told me I should start my own line of lip colors. He loved the colors I had blended and told me if I ever decided to do something with my creative talent he would carry my products in his salon in Bal Harbor. I thanked him for the compliment, and said I would think about it, which I did the entire flight home. I struggled back and forth with this idea and finally figured, why not?

Two weeks later I used my entire life savings, took a major leap of faith, and started my first company, *Lost Art Cosmetics*. I did exactly what he told me I should do, and it was a fantastic experience. My products sold well, and we landed several accounts in Chicago. Just like my stylist friend promised, we landed his account in Bal Harbor and many others in Miami.

It was a wonderful learning experience. I was having the time of my life. In the mid-nineties, fashion was big in Miami and Chicago. I expanded my business. We not only designed lip products, but I also hired several talented artists and started a subsidiary company, *Lost Art Cosmetics Studio*. We organized fashion shows and high-profile events as premier artists and did styling for corporate clients. Business was good.

However, within two years, I'd lost my enthusiasm. I was no longer as eager or focused on my business. It seemed like all I did was run from one social event or party to another. My friends were interested in partying, staying out until all hours of the morning, and mooching off of me as much as they could get away with. My time with these "friends" did not in any way lift me up or encourage my greatness. In fact, I realized when I took an honest look, they were sucking the life out of me. I felt my creativity fade away into bitterness and resentment. Worst of all, I was exhausted.

Breaking Up With "Debbie Downers"

One morning, much earlier than I normally woke up, my grandmother called my house. I didn't make it a practice of answering calls that early but for some reason I did that morning, and I am so glad I did.

When my grandmother asked me how business was going, I could not hide my frustration.

I told her how exhausted, bitter, and inattentive to work I felt. I told her how my friends were a drain and a disappointment, how I was finding it hard to focus or create, and how I no longer enjoyed what I was doing. My grandmother listened carefully as I emptied my basket of woes, and then told me it was time to break up with my friends.

Wait. Break up with my friends? I did not know you could do that.

"Of course you can," she told me. "Call each one of your "friends" that do not contribute in any way to either elevating your cause or supporting you and break up with them."

One thing you must know about my grandmother is she was the wisest woman I have ever known. If she told me to break up with my so-called friends, then that is exactly what I needed to do. If you are lucky, you have a person like my grandmother in your life. I have two; my sister is my other source of wisdom.

When I got off the phone with her, I grabbed my trusty black book. (Yes, black book, this was clearly before cell phones were available.) I went through and circled all the "friends" I had no real connection with. I called everyone who was not an asset to my cause or simply wanted me for what I had to offer but did not contribute in a positive way to my life. And then I took my grandmother's advice. I politely broke up with fifteen people that day and I am not exaggerating.

I cleaned house! I'm sure I confused several of them, but I wished them well and told all of them I needed to stay super focused on my business and to please not call me anymore. I told them I appreciated the time we had together, but I really had to put my energy into my business, and that, as they say, was the end of that!

Today I still take inventory of the people in my life, and I only surround myself with people who I know truly love me and have my best interests in their hearts. The people in my inner circle have been there as cheerleaders as I attempt to conquer one adventure after another and I in turn love doing the same for them.

I am not saying that you have to stop loving family and friends who you still feel attached to, but if they are "Debbie Downers" then you need to really consider reducing the amount of time you give them; or have a serious conversation with them about what you need from them if they want to continue to be a part of your life. Remember you and you alone are responsible for your journey and not the "Debbie Downers" in your life. Surround yourself with only those who you view as an example of who you want to be, those who raise you up and support your journey, and those who show their love in encouraging and supportive ways.

After "cleaning house" I found the act of breaking up with unsupportive friends had cleared enough space for me to create again. I loved spending time to myself and not feeling like I had to go out all of the time. I became particular when it came to sharing my time and space with people.

My environment became peaceful, and I fell in love with my career again. I operated that company for eight years and it was one of the best times of my life. No regrets!

Some of you may think breaking up with friends was a drastic move. And you're right. It was. However, clearing that space and creating calm instead of chaos was the best thing I had done for myself. Truth be told, I did not miss even one of those friends.

Things or Objects That Need to Go!

We live in a country full of opportunity and abundance. So, we tend to chase the next shiny toy as we tire of the previous one. Another act of self-love is letting go of things and habits that are not serving you well. This was hard for me at first. Over time I collected things such as clothing I was so attached to that even when I no longer fit into them anymore, I refused to get rid of them. I had an incredible wardrobe but if I was honest, many pieces had not been worn for years. I kept telling myself I will be a size 0 again so I better hang on to them.

One thing about this Sicilian girl is, as I got older, I developed curves, especially after having three children. I have not been a size 0 since I was in my twenties. Purging my wardrobe for the first time was painful, but once I donated my clothes, within a week I forgot about at least half of the clothes I donated. I only remember two dresses that I wish I still had. Now I make it a habit to purge my closet twice a year. If I haven't worn an outfit that year, it goes bye-bye!

I donate my clothes and things to others who need them. It feels great to help provide for others, and I believe it is our responsibility to contribute to those less fortunate.

Habits That Do Not Serve You Well

When I started writing this book, I was very excited to share it with my ex-husband. He is very supportive, and he really wants to write his own book on Real Estate Law. He's an excellent Attorney and has so much knowledge to share. When I told him how much time I spend writing he was shocked. He told me he wished he had time to write as much as I do. I told him he does have time to write. He corrected himself and said that he knows he needs to *make* the time.

Glued to the News

We went over his typical day and within a 30-second conversation, we came to the agreement that if he stopped watching the news for hours every day and put his cell phone away, he would clear at least four hours a day to write. You can get a lot of writing done in four hours. Scrolling through TikTok, Facebook, and Instagram for several hours a day is not the best use of your time if you are trying to achieve goals in your life that can elevate you.

He is obsessed with the News. He literally has the news on from the time he wakes up until he goes to sleep. He even has it on at his office while he works, and playing in his car when he drives to work.

Breaking that habit will be as painful to him as getting rid of some of my favorite fashion pieces were to me, but once he frees himself of that habit, I am sure he will be extremely happy with the creative space he will make for himself.

Cell Phone Addiction

One day recently I was listening to a motivational audio book. Reading is one of my most favorite things to do, and I try to read or listen to five books a month. I *love* books! The author was sharing statistics of how many times a day the average American picks up their cell phone to check it. The answer was between 120 and 140 times a day! What? I did not believe him, so I counted how many times a day I was grabbing my phone. I quickly recognized that I was grabbing my phone out of habit and checking for texts, emails, *YouTube* videos, and for several other unnecessary reasons. I was one of the statistics! I also noticed I was scanning the Yahoo news feed on my phone several times a day. I hate the news! Why was I doing that? Habit is why I was doing that.

Now I put my phone in my room or in my purse. Unless I need it for work related issues or to check on my kids, I do not pick up my phone. I do not fill my precious time with addictive and needless information that wastes my time and isn't productive. All I can say is freedom from that habit has made me a much more peaceful and productive person.

I give myself 30 minutes at the end of the day if I want to, to check Facebook or other things. As for those news feeds? Those were the first to go!

At least 75% of the crap in the news is not only not newsworthy, but also nasty and horrible examples of the hate and division going on in our country today. Unless it is something that will affect me or my family, I would rather not check in to the crazy. Very seldom is there anything in the news that feeds my soul or contributes to my happiness. I have no doubt that if there is something really important like a wildfire heading our way (or a zombie apocalypse) the people in my life who care about me will let me know in time to take the appropriate action. If I have to know what is going on, I will ask one of the men in my life who does not get emotionally upset watching the news to give me an update. Hands down, defeating cell-phone addiction is one the best things I have done for myself!

See Fear for What It Is

While we're cleaning house, let's get rid of one more useless thing: unreasonable fear. I realize we already talked about this, but I want to touch on it again here because it is extremely important when cleaning up our mental house.

Oxford Languages defines fear as: (noun) An unpleasant emotion caused by the belief that someone or something is dangerous, likely to cause physical or emotional pain, or is a threat; (verb) to be afraid of something or someone, likely to be dangerous or threatening circumstances.

Fear can be an intense and very unpleasant emotion especially in relationship to the unknown.

It is a response to perceiving or recognizing the possibility of dangerous outcomes that can be real or imagined. I hate to say it but most of the fear we feel is attached to imagined outcomes or when we lose control of the outcome. I had no control of my father's choices, and I had no control of my father's outcome, but my biggest fear presented itself when I almost lost my father. We will confront fear more throughout this book:

Remember: Courage can always conquer fear!

Making it Personal

Once again, I invite you to find a safe, quiet space where you can focus your attention on cleaning house. Give yourself some time to dig down deep and think of all of the people who love you and support your greatness. Write them down and show gratitude for their positive influence in your life. Then write down the people who are the Debbie Downers, the people who would rather see you fail than succeed, those who may be so jealous of your talent and potential that they try to sabotage your success. Then, love, honor, and respect *yourself* by breaking up with them!

Next think about all the objects and habits that clutter and complicate your life. What things can you do without? What about unfounded fears? Surely you can let go of some of those.

Make a list of people who have loved you and supported your greatness. Whisper a "Thank you" as an act of gratitude for being a positive influence in your life.

Identify Debbie Downers in your life. People who take your time and energy and give nothing in return. (It's okay. No one's going to judge.)
Now, love, honor, and respect *yourself* by breaking up with them or reducing the amount of time you spend with them.

Now think about objects and habits that clutter and complicate your life and drag you down. Is it time to say bye-bye? Put them on the list.

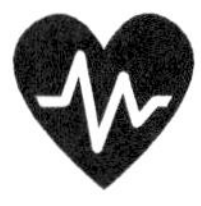

"You grow through what you go through."
~ Author Unknown

Every morning I spend time in prayer and meditation before I get out of bed. I pray for my family and friends, this country, the condition of this world, those in need, and I show God gratitude for the life He has gifted me. I am a Christian and prayer keeps me connected to God which in turn helps me understand, without fear, what is going on in this world and why. I study the Bible daily and I also meditate and do deep breathing exercises to calm my body, slow down my mind and help get me focused on what I need to do each day. These are acts of self-care that are just as important to me as hitting the gym first thing in the morning or eating healthy.

That is me and my beliefs. I understand and respect that religion is not for everyone. Other faiths, religions, and beliefs should be respected, and no one should be shamed or ridiculed for what they do or do not believe in. That leads to hate and division and isn't there enough of that in the world?

Although it sounds like it, my life is not perfect. I use colorful words sometimes and Lord knows I am flawed just like everyone else. I joke that God has me on a retractable leash. When I stray too far, He reels me back in, puts me back in my place and then sends me out to conquer another day. I know without a doubt that every day when I pray it builds my faith and creates a fierceness in me that keeps me focused on the important things that I must do to keep myself, my family, and my company thriving.

Whatever your faith is, it is important to have a spiritual connection that feeds your mind, body, and soul. A spiritual connection keeps us grounded and helps hold us accountable. We live in a country where anxiety, stress, and uncertainty have become the normal. Suicide is at an all-time high. According to Health Watch and CBS News 2023, nearly 1 in 3 adolescents are being treated for mental health issues. According to The American Psychological Association, in 2023, 1 in 5 teenagers have seriously considered suicide in the United States. Teens are not the only concern. Suicide in adults has increased at alarming rates with men being 4 times more likely to commit suicide than women. Mental health has become a primary concern in the US. As of 2023 almost 1 in 4 people are taking prescription drugs for mental health issues such as depression, anxiety, and extreme stress.

The aftermath of the Covid-19 pandemic left a lot of Americans without the mental health care that many people needed but were unable to access due to such a large demand on mental health care providers and not enough mental health care professionals to manage the high demand. Being home with your kids, spouses, and families 24-7, loss of jobs, and financial devastation pushed many people past their breaking point. There was a major increase in the use of drugs and alcohol to self soothe and the uncertainty, media scare tactics, and political manipulation took a serious toll on Americans.

A rise in violent crimes, a broken economy, and political hate and division has caused people to pass judgement and be hateful towards others that they do not even know. Divorce is at a record high leaving a path of destruction for our young people to clean up. Most homes do not have strong parental partnerships. Many of our youth live in single parent homes leaving children confused and angry and parents frustrated, overworked, and struggling. If there was ever a time to lean into your faith it is now. I thank God every day for the safety, security, and guidance that my faith offers. It has been a life saver for me. Literally!

Humans have souls, which means we have a need for some kind of spiritual understanding. I was born Catholic, then drifted into having no faith at all, before becoming a Christian. I remember when I was angry and Agnostic, with no boundaries, and no understanding of why I was here or what my purpose was on this earth. I was self-serving, and I was self-centered. I really did not like the person I was back then. When I became a Christian, my anger softened and turned into curiosity which led me to being open to learn and understand God's will and purpose for me. Now I am living my life serving others because that is my purpose. A purpose I am proud of and a purpose that my God loving and God-fearing grandmother made my sister and I fully understand before she left this earth. My faith may not be for everyone and that is ok, but it is for me. I could not imagine my life without Jesus.

Everyone is different and has their own set of beliefs. It is in my opinion that the more you are connected spiritually, the world tends to be less scary as we navigate each day.

Prayer vs. Meditation

Is prayer and meditation the same thing? Some people will say that prayer is their meditation, and I have heard people say meditation is their way of praying. I see them as two different things. When I pray it is purposeful and directed to God and is my way of building a bond and relationship with Him. I worship through prayer, and I go to God when I am grateful, or I need help and guidance. My faith is my relationship and expression for the love I have for God as a Christian woman. He is my spiritual connection to something much greater than myself that keeps me accountable for my actions, gives me a strong moral compass, provides peace and love, and helps me to understand the purpose and meaning of my life.

Meditation is a tool I use to calm my body, go into a deep relaxation, and focus myself on my agenda for the day. I use it to re-center my mind if I get too distracted. That is the wonderful thing about meditation. It is an especially useful tool that helps clear the clutter, allowing for creative space in our minds. Meditating in a relaxing way benefits both the mind and the body. I have used meditation to help me overcome and identify emotional obstacles from past pain and trauma and then I use prayer to ask God to help guide me to find forgiveness, give me patience, and have a gentleness of heart. I rely on God's strength to overcome those challenges.

When people tell me that having a spiritual connection is not for everyone, I strongly disagree. The emotional, mental, and physical benefits of having some kind of spiritual connection far outweigh managing life and its challenges alone. Research shows that people with some kind of spiritual connection tend to be emotionally and mentally healthier, possibly even living longer as well.

If you look at the most successful athletes in the world, almost every one of them uses prayer, meditation, or visualization meditation techniques to condition themselves and prepare them for their sport. Many of the most successful businesses people in the world as well as many celebrities have some kind of spiritual connection, many thanking God for their success or crediting their success on the habitual practice of meditation. You cannot expect to take on the weight of the world without giving your mind and spirit the help they need to achieve the greatness you were meant for. Otherwise, you will turn to other people in your life to navigate your emotional, spiritual, and mental health. That is not a fair expectation of others, and more importantly, it is a huge disservice to yourself.

When people work out, they spend an hour or so in the gym. They work all areas of their body to strengthen and keep it healthy. Why would you not do the same for the mental, emotional, and spiritual side of your being? Your mental health is just as important as any other part of your body, and it needs constant care just like the rest of your body. Through meditation, prayer, or both, you have an opportunity to connect with yourself in a way that only you can. Meditation and prayer are a true act of radical self-love. (I will tell you more about Radical Self-Love in the next chapter.)

The other thing I love about meditation and prayer is that it is motivational, it costs absolutely nothing, is extremely powerful, and is at my disposal whenever I need it. No one can take it from me. I can meditate or pray anywhere at any time, and it can change my mood and disposition quickly. I do not have to have a dreadful day. I can change that in minutes. I can use it to re-focus when I feel I am getting distracted and anyone who knows me knows I am off chasing butterflies a lot. So, meditation, especially, is a necessary tool for those of us who are easily distracted.

When you neglect your emotional, mental, and spiritual health, you pawn your happiness off on others by default, trying to make them responsible for your journey. Your journey is meant for you to navigate and not for someone else to. They have their own journey to navigate. You are accountable for your choices. They are accountable for their choices.

Some people make others responsible for the direction their life has taken so they do not have to take responsibility when things go wrong. That is not only self-destructive behavior, but it leads to unfulfilled expectations of others, and will destroy your relationships because you expect others to be responsible for you and clean up your messes, which is frankly a cop out. I see this all the time in marriages, friendships, and parental/family relationships. It is co-dependent behavior, and it is very unhealthy.

We all know that person, family member, or friend where everything in their life is in shambles, it is always someone else's fault, and they are always the victim. They never take responsibility for their choices, behavior, or circumstances. It is unfortunate but you cannot be their savior. They need to navigate their own journey, and you need to be clear with them and set boundaries if you still want a relationship with these types of personalities.

Meditation Lets you Time Travel

Really? Absolutely. Let's go back for a moment to my story about the Stringy-Blonde-Haired-Girl.

When you are injured emotionally as a little kid, the incident is in your past, but all the hurts, fears, obstacles, and doubts keep popping up in your present, consciously and subconsciously. A therapist can help you identify these areas if you feel you need additional support. For example, say a person pushed you down and you became fearful. Those fears can keep manifesting in the choices you make throughout your life.

What the therapist cannot do is go back in time and clean that space out for you. They can guide you, but you must do the work. Honestly, nothing anyone else can say to you can help you unless you are willing to do the work yourself.

This is where meditation comes in as an effective tool. With meditation, you can go back into yourself, go back to that child who was traumatized or that little girl who was pushed down on the playground. You can visualize through meditation that you hug her, pick her up, and give her the love she really deserves. This is where I go back to my little girl and tell her how much I love her, tell her how incredible she is, and that God gave her life great purpose and put that Stringy-Blonde-Haired Girl "ghost" to rest.

Some of you might be saying, "But Christen, my life has been nothing but a series of failures. I have nothing to offer that little child." Let me repeat what I said earlier in this book. Every one of us harbors a better version of ourselves deep down. I am not saying you are harboring a perfect person, but you certainly are not a worthless human who has no purpose. You may be off track right now, but you always have wisdom and value; you just have not manifested it yet. Meditation starts with desire and that is all it takes to begin to build a better life. Meditation and prayer can help you focus your desire to live a better life.

Gratitude Meditation

Whatever your faith, religion, or belief system might be, it is important to express gratitude for the things that bring peace, joy, and beauty into your life. A beautiful sky, a call from a friend at just the right time, each day you have been gifted. If you have ever watched the TV program "My 600 Pound Life," you have learned people need a reason to fight for their lives. These people are going up against the impossible. One of the first steps in their journey is always recognizing areas where they can express gratitude in their life. As they fight through obstacles on their journey, they become grateful for all the things they took for granted before they lost their health, like the physical freedom to take a walk outside or attend a social event. They begin to live again. They start to see the greater version of themselves coming to the surface. It is inspiring.

The show always starts with a recognition that there is a spirit inside a person that is willing to fight for their life. The reason they are willing to fight is they have identified something they see worth holding on to, something to be grateful for. There is always something that somebody can be grateful for, or they would not be here today, they would have given up.

Maybe you have a family member who needs you, or a dream you never realized because your size is holding you back. Maybe you are grateful for a wake up call that sets you back on the path to working on your health. Having gratitude triggers the brain to refocus on the positive instead of the negative and is another example of radical self-love.

Becoming Unbreakable

I love this feeling. Feeling unbreakable. I have learned through meditation and prayer that I possess the power to be unbreakable. I did not know I had it in me, and the realization came as a bit of a surprise.

Over the last five years, especially as our world started changing so dramatically, I noticed I was feeling uncertainty from the pandemic, and the political climate that has spewed so much hate and division. It was affecting my heart, my hope, my faith, and my thoughts about me and my children's future.

I suffered a lot of loss during that time. Many people I knew either died or were severely impacted by Covid-19. I stepped away from meditation and my faith and my heart and spirit suffered. It did not take long for me to figure out that I needed to re-connect spiritually and clear that fear.

As soon as I started taking better care of my spiritual and mental health again, I reminded myself that in the face of challenges outside of my control, the one thing I *can* control is how I view those challenges. I can switch gears, lean into my faith, and redirect that energy wasted on fear and turn it towards problem solving.

I stopped watching the news and eliminated that crazy ride of hatred and division and when I started praying for hope and love instead, the fear disappeared. It was simply no longer my focus. Hope and love became my focus and after staying consistent in my faith, my attitude changed. I started noticing and attracting more hope and love in my environment and community.

As I mentioned before in *Chapter 4, Facing our Fears*, it is useless to fear the things that we cannot control. I had to remind myself of that. To become unbreakable, you must control the source of your love, hope, and purpose.

I allowed myself to grieve for those I lost. It was painful. However, I also protected my emotional, mental, and spiritual space so I would not be broken by everything going on around me during those challenging times. I believe that through prayer and meditation, I can protect and strengthen my emotional, mental, and spiritual wellbeing.

I do not believe in chance or coincidence. I believe everything happens for a reason and we are where we are when we need to be there. I believe in the law of attraction and the power of prayer. Have faith, open your mind and the spirit within you and show gratitude toward your God and your place in the intricate, incredible weave of the universe.

Do not allow yourself to be pulled into garbage and useless crap that sucks the life out of you. Do not worry about trying to fit into a broken world. This is your journey. You create your own path to your happiness.

Why are you Grateful?

As I just mentioned, the world we live in can be scary at times. It's easy to focus on things that bring you down, make you fearful, rob you of peace. Whether it is the political climate, or something happening closer to home, you can be overwhelmed by negative input. But there is also great beauty and grace in our world.

Everybody has at least one person, one thing, or place they can be grateful for. Just go outside and look around. Is the sky blue today? Be grateful.

Guided Meditations

If prayer is not your thing and if you have never done any kind of meditation before, you might be thinking, "But Christen, I have no idea how to even start a meditation." Never fear! The Internet is a great place to start. Search YouTube for "Guided Meditations" and you will discover dozens of them, including meditation for gratitude, better sleep, and deep relaxation. For Christians, there are some beautiful Christian meditations and prayers. (I use YouTube meditations every day.) You can also download mediation and prayer Apps to your Smart Phone. I have also provided a list of suggested meditations in the Resources section at the back of this book.

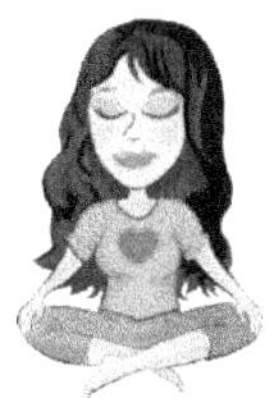

Once you have found an appropriate guided meditation, find yourself a quiet, comfortable place and sit cross legged or lie down on your back. You may find using a sleep mask helps to shut out distractions. Now, start the guided meditation and just listen and do as the guide tells you. You'll be amazed how you feel afterward.

Making it Personal

Take a moment in a quiet space to write down the people and things in your world you are grateful for, even if it is nothing more than the sun shining today, or your shoes are right where you left them next to the bed.

JOURNAL

Make a list of the things you are grateful for, even if you are having a difficult day. Take time and really focus on that gratitude.

____

____

____

____

____

____

____

____

Now think of times in the past when Young You could have used some love and support. During meditation, give your younger, less experienced self some love and care through that experience.

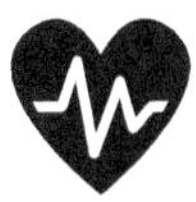

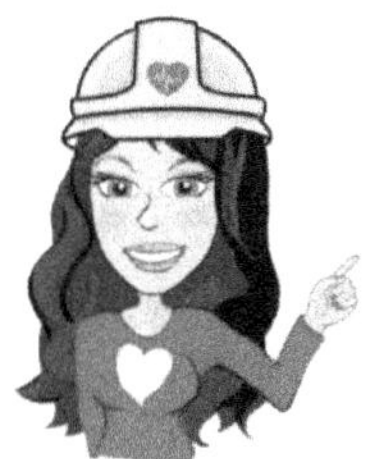

RED FLAG WARNING: This is a very sensitive subject for me. I'm going put on my hard hat and go on a rant now, but I promise you, it's for a good cause. You need to put your metaphorical hard hat on too, because this is not going to be an easy chapter to read.

I get really frustrated (and to be honest, pissed off) when I read or hear people talking about Radical Self-Love in the context of accepting and loving your body no matter what your size. Really? Tell that to my clients who are 400 pounds plus with one foot in the grave who struggle just to function day-to-day. When certain celebrities and the media spread the message of Radical Self-Love by telling you to accept and love your morbidly obese body, we need to be honest about what that looks like in its entirety, because it is more than just accepting the body you live in.

Loving yourself as you are is not about the way you look. It encompasses the way you love and care for your mind, body, and soul in its entirety. Let me say this again… True expression of Self-Love is the way you love and care for your mind, body, and spirit in its entirety!

First of all, beauty is in the eye of the beholder. This chapter has nothing to do with the concept of beauty by society's standards. So, haters, do not misconstrue what I am saying here. Beauty has nothing to do with your size.

I support loving the skin you are in. I support loving your body when you are working to improve your health no matter what your size. Let me emphasize, it is an act of self-love to take care of the body you were given.

I support loving your body whether you are short, tall, stocky, small boned, big boned, black skin, brown skin, yellow skin, white skin, long hair, short hair, or no hair at all. I support loving yourself when you are born with mental or physical limitations or if you have experienced trauma that has thrown life-changing mental or physical limitations at you. All of this I support 100%.

However, when being overweight or obese puts your health at risk or means you must take prescription medications because of your lifestyle choices, I do not call that Self-Love. I understand the message the media is trying to project and in a perfect world. If 74.6 % of the US population were not in the midst of a major health crisis and obesity epidemic, then we could have a self-love fest all day long.

Unfortunately, that is not the country we live in. To-day, the United States is considered the unhealthiest country in the world! According to the *World Population Review*, America is the unhealthiest country globally because of its high obesity rate and the lifestyle illnesses associated with excessive weight gain.

What are lifestyle illnesses associated with obesity in the US? Here is a reminder: cardiovascular disease, heart attacks, stroke, high blood pressure, type-2 diabetes, high cholesterol, peripheral arterial disease, chronic inflammatory diseases, and some cancers to name just a few. Can you see that we are in a critical health crisis?

Obesity alone is a serious epidemic killing Americans at alarming rates. I am willing to fall on my sword for this one and I will continue to scream from the mountain tops if I must that this epidemic must change because the percentage of obesity in America just keeps growing and growing and people are dying all in the name of the Standard American Diet!

In 2022, according to the CDC, Harvard Medical and the National Institutes of Health:

- 74.6% of Americans are in the overweight, obese, morbidly obese, and severe morbidly obese categories. Yes, now they have added a new obese category in the medical community. (Severe morbidly obese).

- 43% are in the obese category (BMI 30 – 35).

- 10% are in the morbidly obese category (BMI 40+) and severe morbidly obese (BMI 40-100+).

- The Obesity rate has tripled since the 1960's from 13 to 43% and doubled in the last 10 years.

- The #1 cause of death in the United States is heart attack in both men and women.

- The CDC stated in 2022 that in the last 5 years, there has been a 35% increase in the number of people taking anti-depressants.

According to the CDC, obesity related conditions including heart disease, stroke, type-2 diabetes, and certain types of cancer are among the leading causes of preventable premature deaths in the United States.

According to the National Institutes of Health, obesity is among the leading causes of elevated cardiovascular disease.

According to the World Health Organization, the most important behavioral risk factor of heart disease and stroke is an unhealthy diet and physical inactivity. Also, the number one pharmaceutical sold in the U.S. is for high blood pressure due to lifestyle choices.

According to the Association of Clinical Endocrinologist (AACE), obesity has now been renamed in the medical community as Adiposity-Based Chronic Disease.

I could go on and on with a multitude of alarming statistics. So, please stop referring to the term Radical Self-Love as loving the body you are in regardless of size. It is clearly much more than that.

Radical self-love is only fully expressed when you love and care for yourself, body, mind, and spirit. You cannot say you love yourself and not take care of the body, mind, and spirit you have been given. If you do not take care of your physical being are you expressing self-love? It is not possible to let your health and body deteriorate while you are eating the foods that make you unhealthy and are killing you, then call that Radical Self-Love. It is self-destruction, not self-love.

When you take steps of any kind to better your health and reduce the risk of lifestyle-associated disease, that's when you are expressing Radical Self-Love.

Redefining Radical Self-Love

We have talked about what Radical Self-Love is NOT. Now let's see some examples of what Radical Self-Love IS, especially as it relates to your body. Your size does not matter. You are expressing Radical Self-Love when:

- You take action steps toward changing the foods you put in your body to nutrient-dense foods that will cleanse and heal your body.

- You get active and moving to ensure a healthier cardiovascular system.

- You get the quality sleep your body needs to restore itself.

- You drink the recommended amount of water to stay hydrated.

- You minimize your alcohol intake.

- You eliminate sugar, artificial sweeteners, and simple carbohydrates from your diet.

- You reduce your saturated fat intake to 5% daily (the average American eats 33%).

- You reduce your stress by practicing meditation and mindfulness.

- You take time to meditate, pray, or care for your emotional, mental, and spiritual health.

- You surround yourself with people who want to see you succeed and support your journey back to good health.

- You educate yourself about the most wholistic and natural ways to care for your body.

- You steer clear of toxic people and negative influences such as news or mindless online content.

- You read or listen to audiobooks that educate and motivate you to be the best version of yourself.

- You consult with a mental healthcare provider, therapist, or psychologist if you struggle and need additional support.

Forget the Media Hype

This is where we've all been duped. The media is not concerned about your health. All this talk about loving the body you're in gives morbidly obese people a reason to stay that way or get even bigger. That's not Radical Self-Love. If you are overweight, and your blood pressure is great, your glucose numbers are normal and your cholesterol is in the normal range, and you are not on prescription meds to manage any of those things, then by all means, embrace yourself, and embrace your body. You have beaten the odds.

However, I work every day with people who are obese and morbidly obese, and I'm here to tell you, there are very few human beings who are morbidly obese whose numbers are in the healthy range. The media's *Big is Beautiful* message not only condones unhealthy lifestyle, but it also feeds the pocketbooks of our agricultural, food, and big pharma industries. What our advertisers are actually promoting when they bombard us with fast food commercials is a risky, unhealthy lifestyle.

Here's what this message is really saying: "Embrace heart disease, type-2 diabetes, and stroke."

When you travel to Europe and walk the streets of Italy for example, it only takes a moment to see the rest of the world isn't jumping on that bandwagon.

Let's look at another aspect: When the Radical Self-Love movement focuses on beauty as the goal, many people choose to do anything, including taking pills, trying numerous aesthetic procedures, or even having plastic surgery to achieve it. Instead of focusing on health, we see people substituting prescriptions and supplements for healthy nutrition. When people are focused on their appearance, they can neglect their physical health because they don't think of health from the inside out.

Understand this: Accepting obesity no matter how beautiful, how famous, or what prescriptions you can take to counteract the symptoms, will cut your life short. Without a healthy inside, the outside cannot maintain its natural beauty.

According to the Bariatric Centers of America, Obesity shortens life expectancy in individuals with moderate obesity (30 to 35 BMI) by three years, while patients with severe obesity (40+ BMI) may take ten or more years off their life. (The average life expectancy currently is 80.2 for women and 74.8 for men.)

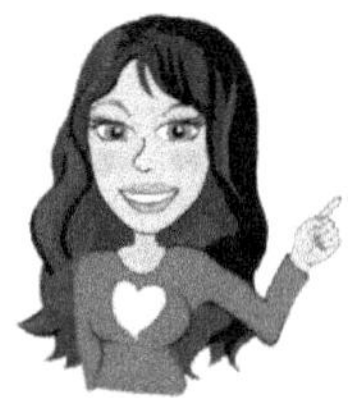

We've shot ourselves in the foot here in the United States trivializing obesity. Men and women are getting bigger and bigger. In twenty years of working with my clients, I've never had one single person seeking help for lifestyle disease and obesity come to me and say, "I feel absolutely amazing in the skin I'm in," or "I'm okay being overweight, I just want to get healthy."

The truth is their self-image, and their emotional state have taken massive hits because of their size. They are worn down and tired of carrying all that weight. They are ready to do anything to reverse the damage their lifestyle disease has created.

When I was heavier, I hated to go shopping. Every time I tried something on, I was disgusted when I looked in the mirror. I would walk out of the dressing room choking back tears. I couldn't fit into the clothes I wanted, and clothes that fit didn't look like what I thought they would when they were on me. There was never one day when I looked in the mirror said "God, I look great." These days, I'm happy in my skin because I've done the work and I've lost the extra weight, but most importantly I have regained my health, and I can tell you, nothing tastes as good as healthy feels!

We have this huge population of people who are morbidly obese with one foot in the grave, and we keep feeding them body positivity messages. How about feeding them encouraging messages that build their self-confidence to get them healthy again.

Luxury Sports Car or Jalopy?

When you're born, you are given one vehicle to drive you through your life. Because I'm Italian, I choose to be a Ferrari. That Ferrari must get me from point A in my journey to point Z. From the beginning of my life to the end.

Am I going to drive that Ferrari into a tree? No. Of course not. Am I going to put peanut butter in the gas tank? Am I going to drive that Ferrari around on a flat tire? No, and no. I want to be able to take my Ferrari out on the open road and enjoy the beauty and the power of owning such a fine-tuned machine. I'm going to keep it polished, make sure it gets regular maintenance, and top-grade fuel. I'm going to keep my Ferrari in beautiful condition so I can continue to drive it to the end of my journey. Who knows, my Ferrari may even go up in value.

I cannot buy a new vehicle, lease a new vehicle, or rent a different model. We are given only one. Is this resonating with you? You can drive a fine, functional, beautiful vehicle that you can enjoy driving all your life or you can drive a beat-up jalopy that breaks down constantly, is running on flat tires, and needs an overwhelming amount of tedious and expensive maintenance.

You have a choice about how you take care of the body you were born with so it can serve you well till the end of your days. Do you want to be driving a Ferrari through life, or are you willing to accept an old beat-up jalopy? Radical Self-Love is taking care of that body and honoring the gift you were born with.

In America, the media and the food and drug industries are all peddling jalopies right now. How do we know? Think about it. If over three quarters of a country's population is unhealthy, we're doing something wrong. Pushing the "embracing-the-body-you-are-in" message isn't making people feel better about themselves. It's ruining their health.

Skinny Fat

Let's not leave out another segment of the population: The "skinny fat." This population is what is technically known as Normal Weight Obesity. It is the condition of having normal body weight but with a high body fat percentage. Just because someone might be of normal body weight does not mean they are healthy. Normal Weight Obesity can affect up to 34% of the population in the normal weight category.

These people are equally at risk for all the same life-style diseases that the obesity categories are. The only difference is most of them do not know it.

As a Medical Exercise Specialist, I had many clients in the normal weight category who had ridiculously high blood pressure and high cholesterol. They would often say to me their high blood pressure or high cholesterol was hereditary. They would blame it on their mom or dad and never take into consideration that the foods they were eating were putting them at risk for serious medical conditions.

The Price of Denial

One of those clients happened to become a good friend. He trained with me twice a week and we argued constantly about nutrition. One day I patiently waited for Frank to come for his training session, and he never showed up. I called him, but he never answered. The next week the same thing happened. Finally, I looked up his address and went to his house. When I arrived, I saw his family members packing up a moving truck full of his furniture and personal belongings. I was surprised that he would be moving without telling me. I spoke to his sister who looked extremely distraught. She told me that Frank had passed away a few weeks before from a stroke. They found him passed out on a trail where he used to run.

His cholesterol level was off the charts. He lived for a few days after the stroke, but his body gave out and he died without being able to say goodbye to his family. This broke my heart. Frank ran five miles a day so he could keep his weight down but ate all the crap food he wanted thinking he was safe. Frank was 42 years old when he died.

While I stood there reflecting on how preventable his death could have been, his sister went into the house and came back with a brand-new book she said he had just purchased. It was "The China Study" on plant-based nutrition. She gave it to me, and said she knew Frank would want me to have it. I still have that book.

Skinny Fat Girl

I have another client who easily fits into size two skinny jeans. She told me she had just been diagnosed with a non-alcoholic fatty liver. This can be every bit as life threatening as the effects of obesity. She had no idea she was at risk. So, how did this happen? Food! The Standard American diet! She knew her cholesterol was high, but she did not associate any of the symptoms she was experiencing with having excessive fat. Her visceral fat was suffocating her liver and once that happened her liver would die if she didn't take immediate action and change. You cannot live without your liver. It has a very important job to do: processing blood and breaking down nutrients and chemicals that your blood then carries throughout the body. The liver regulates most of the chemicals in your blood, then filters the nutrients into the blood stream and waste is excreted as a byproduct called bile. Once the bile has served its purpose, these waste products ultimately leave your body as feces. Every organ in your body serves a purpose.

While a very small percentage of people with fatty liver disease have a genetic predisposition, the majority of people got there because they've been eating the Standard American Diet.

I had been living under the assumption I was in great health. My cholesterol was high, but I was normal weight with low blood pressure and I was a Master Swimmer. Then I was diagnosed with non-alcoholic fatty liver disease. What a shock! My doctor said I could control it with diet and exercise, but I had been doing that all along, cutting back on sugar, alcohol, and red meats, exercising every day. Obviously, that wasn't the answer. What I had failed to do was add back in the nutrient-rich foods my body needed to heal and maintain the proper balance.

It took only 6 weeks on Christen's nutrient-rich, whole foods plan to bring my liver panel numbers back to normal. I am so grateful and have made this a permanent lifestyle change.
K. Larcomb

The bottom line is it's up to you to wade through all the hype and pop culture jargon and look at what is really important to maintaining or reclaiming your health. We can't go on like this. Something has to change. If our government and media and the people who feed us and run our healthcare systems won't take responsibility to turn the obesity epidemic around, who does that leave to take responsibility? You!

It's time to put on your big girl (or big boy) pants and take an *honest* look in that mirror. What I want you to realize is that if you are unhealthy, taking several medications every day just to keep yourself alive, it doesn't matter what you look like. You are at risk for the top killers in the country: Heart attack, type-2 diabetes, high blood pressure, and stroke.

What you should be saying to yourself isn't "Big Is Beautiful" *or* "Love me where I am," or "I hate myself because I'm fat." What you should be saying to that beautiful, worthy, loved person in the mirror is "I'm unhealthy," then answer the question, "What will I do today to fix that?"

If you want a beautiful functioning engine purring under your hood for the rest of your life, then you have to take care of your vehicle.

This is the point I am trying to make: No one else is responsible for your health. It's not easy, but it's not complicated either. Either you take care of the body you're given, or it quits on you and leaves you in a ditch by the side of the road.

The good news is, it's never too late to tune up your engine, pump up those tires, and get yourself back on track. The bad news is most people who want to lose weight and improve their overall health haven't a clue where to start. (That's why I wrote this book.)

Self-Love is an Essential Part in Finding Your Purpose

I told you in the beginning, the Self-Love part would be difficult. Let's face it: We all need a little help in that department. The list I gave you earlier in this chapter is a great place to start. Every single thing on that list is showing yourself Radical Self-Love.

However, there is also a really important thing I deliberately left off the list because I felt it deserved its own chapter, and that is doing the work to find purpose in your life. We'll start work on that in the next chapter.

To finish up this chapter let's take a look at the ways you can show yourself Radical Self-Love.

Making it Personal

Find a quiet place where you can spend some time thinking about the ways you can show yourself Radical Self-Love.

JOURNAL

Review the list I shared earlier in this chapter. What things can you start to do right now? Can you think of any other ways specific to your individual experience? Write them down.

____

____

____

____

____

____

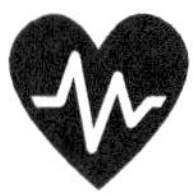

What is the purpose of our life here on earth? My grandmother told me there are two things people chase relentlessly in life: Purpose and Love. She was willing to help me find my purpose, but she said, "You are on your own where love is concerned because the heart wants what the heart wants." She wouldn't advise me on who I should or should not love. She also told me our greatest life lessons come from who we choose to love. I was young when she told me this, so I didn't give it much thought, but as I got older, I came to understand the wisdom in her words.

I was twenty-five when I started to learn what my purpose was. I was living in Chicago working two jobs. I loved one of them, the other I knew was not my life's calling. As it turned out, both jobs taught me helpful skill sets I would rely on later in my journey.

In my twenties I worked hard as a makeup artist for fashion shows and photoshoots, and also as a server at a restaurant. Fashions shows were exciting, and it was great money when the work was there. I was still doing some modeling at the time, again not consistent, so the server job helped fill in to make ends meet. I was having fun though and enjoying my twenties for the most part. I was fearless and just trying to figure life out.

One day I got a phone call from my grandmother inviting me to Thanksgiving at her house in Sarasota, Florida. My heart swelled with anticipation, as I assumed everyone in the family received the same invitation. My family was scattered all over the United States, so these family gatherings were rare.

I arrived in Sarasota Thanksgiving morning prepared for some good ole' home-cooked meals (no one could cook better than my grandmother) and excited to see everyone. I'd been working hard in Chicago, and I was ready for some fun along with hopefully, some much needed relaxation and pampering from my grandmother.

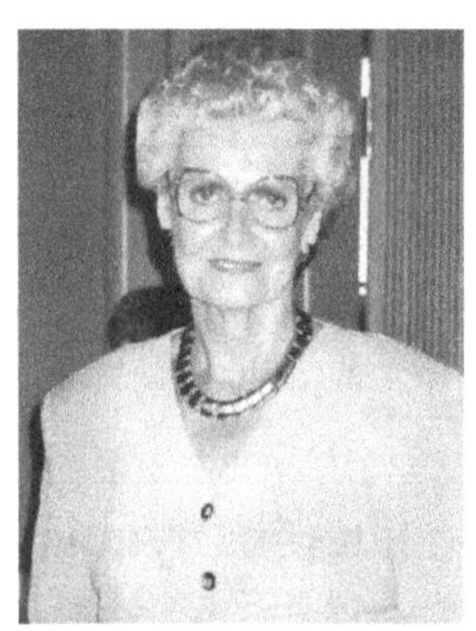

My Grams

I stepped off the plane, made my way to baggage claim, and there she was! (You have to know, my grandmother was very hard to miss. She was six-foot tall and stunning!) My excitement boiled up inside me and then flagged when I scanned the surrounding area and did not recognize anyone else. Of course, I was happy to see her, but I was hoping other members of my family would be there to surprise me, too. I ran to her, and she wrapped me in one of her long-anticipated grandmother's hugs. She always smelled like jasmine, and her hugs always made me feel so safe and loved.

We gathered my suitcases, headed for her car, and as I piled into the front passenger seat I wondered when everyone else would arrive. That's when she hit me with the news: No other family members were coming to Thanksgiving!

What? Nobody else was coming? As you can imagine, I was very disappointed but at the same time I felt honored that she invited me and that we would have some great quality time together. I didn't know what to say. We sat in silence for a few minutes and then, as she drove us back to her house, she asked me an unexpected question: "Chris, do you know what your purpose is?"

I thought about it for a minute and was surprised to find my mind was completely blank. *Was this a trick question?* I stared at her face for a moment, looking for clues in her expression, until she simply asked me the question again.

I shook my head, realizing the truth. "No grams... I do not."

She smiled and said, "Today you are going to learn the purpose of your life."

By the time we arrived at her house my head was spinning with all the possible ways I could learn the purpose of my life on Thanksgiving Day alone with my grandmother. Knowing her, I was about to find out.

I walked in the front door of her house, set my bag down in the entry, and my jaw dropped to the floor. A long table stretched from the entrance of her living room all the way through the dining room. There must have been about fifty chairs lined up on either side. Without explanation, she simply told me "Go put your suitcase in the spare bedroom, change into some comfortable clothes, and meet me in the kitchen."

I did what she asked and after getting out of the super cute dress I was wearing; I put on a comfortable blouse and a pair of jeans and met her in the kitchen.

A Lesson of a Lifetime

The smell of Thanksgiving dinner hit me immediately the moment I walked in and my stomach started growling. I had never seen so much food. It was everywhere! My grandmother always cooked a kick-ass Thanksgiving dinner, but this was a feast like no other. She had a nice-sized kitchen, and every inch of that kitchen was covered with bowls and platters of traditional Thanksgiving delicacies. There were huge turkey trays, tureens of stuffing, piles of greens, mountains of mashed potatoes, and every aroma and dish transported me to the Thanksgivings of my childhood, especially when she started making her secret recipe for the turkey gravy.

When I finally emerged from my journey down memory lane I had to ask, "Grams, I am really confused. I thought you said no one from our family was coming. There are at least fifty chairs around the table. What is going on?"

She gave me a serious look. "You and I are serving fifty homeless people and seniors who have nowhere to go for Thanksgiving. I have been busting my butt in this kitchen for the last three days." Then she went back to stirring the gravy and went on, "You and I are going to serve each and every one of our guests and make sure they have the best Thanksgiving possible. You will not sit down until the last one is served." Then she paused, looked up from the pot and asked, "Any questions?"

Knowing my grandmother, that was not actually an invitation to ask questions. That was the end of that conversation.

We had just a few hours to set the table and get the food and beverages laid out for everyone. It was the hardest work I had ever done and somehow it had become the most rewarding. After feeding fifty complete strangers, most of them homeless, I sat down to eat with them. Everyone at the table was laughing and talking amongst each other. You would have never known that most of these people were strangers with no home to go to. At the far end of the table my grandmother just sat watching people enjoying themselves as they filled their bellies with the same delicious foods she had prepared for me when I was younger. I knew how blessed and appreciative each and every one of these people felt because I felt it too.

After several hours of celebrating Thanksgiving, everyone had finally left, and the house was peaceful once again. My grandmother and I buckled down and got to cleaning the dishes. She packed up what little leftovers remained and put them in a box to donate to her church. After everything was clean and put back in place where it belonged, my grandmother asked me if I would like some tea. Once again, knowing her well, that meant we were going to have a conversation. At last, we were going to have some time alone and I welcomed that. She brought us both a cup of tea and she sat in her favorite chair, and I sat in an identical chair opposite her, with just a small table between us. She looked at me, smiled and asked, "How was your day?"

Piecing the day together in my mind I had to admit, "It was fantastic! Exhausting, but fantastic!"

She stood up and pulled me out of my chair, wrapped me in her arms, and gave me one of her famous hugs. "Now you know your purpose. You are a servant to others. You were called to serve people in whatever capacity your heart takes you. You will never have to chase your purpose again."

I shook my head. "But, Grams, why did you choose me and not any of the other kids in our family?"

"Because you are a survivor, you will always find the answers to your questions, and you have a deep seeded love for others that God planted deep inside your heart." She sat back down and sipped her tea in the way she always did, then put down the cup and fixed me with her serious Grams look. "Being a servant to others is an honorable job. It takes unconditional love and care for people even if you do not like them. I see that in you. God sees that in you. You are a servant."

I went to bed that night completely exhausted, emotionally, mentally, and physically. This was not the Thanksgiving I had envisioned. It turned out to be far greater than that. I felt like I had taken the next step into adulthood and that my journey was about to take a new turn. I went back to Chicago with a new understanding and a fire under my ass to learn more about my purpose. I soon began to realize that my journey and my purpose were merging into parallel paths.

We Were Meant to Evolve

Our mental and emotional growth are a part of our past, present, and future; the natural, evolutionary process that is our life-long journey. Life experiences give us opportunities to make choices that continue this evolution to discover our purpose and our personal greatness. If we make the right choices, we move closer to our greatness, if we make the wrong choices, it is like taking two steps forward and three steps back. However, even making mistakes and wrong choices can create opportunities for a great learning experience and the growth that comes from that.

As my grandmother taught me, we were not put on this earth to remain stagnant. We were put here to go on a journey to learn, evolve, and find our purpose. I was very fortunate to have found my purpose at a very young age, thanks to my grandmother who was so generous with her time and advice to help me find it.

Also, like she told me, the clues to finding my purpose had always been there in my life. They are there in your life, too, if you take a moment to remember. As you grew from a toddler to an adolescent, you slowly became an individual with your own interests and imagination, driving your activities toward what you enjoyed. Unfortunately for all of us, the day comes when a certain experience causes a pivotal shift in our lives, and we realize for the first time there is something wrong in the world or something wrong with us.

Some of our natural talents and gifts can become repressed when hurtful things happen. Those painful circumstances become bigger issues than what we are equipped to manage on our own as kids. These things, left unresolved, can follow us for a very long time and drag us horribly off the course to finding our purpose. This is where healing from past experiences is necessary if you want to move forward. Past trauma can paralyze us emotionally and stunt our emotional development if we do not heal some of those past wounds.

Releasing the Past

Releasing the past is a necessary process as I have mentioned a few times. You *can* go back and heal past wounds. I know this from personal experience. First, however, you need to be willing to acknowledge what it is that is holding you back.

We talked about this in *Chapter 6, Meditation/Prayer*, and you may have written down an experience in your journal.

If that experience is not something you can identify on your own, you may need to have a therapist help you.

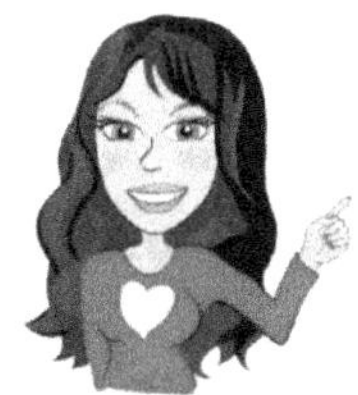

If you do not already have a mental health care provider, check the RESOURCES section in the back of this book for a place to start.

As you revisit these past circumstances, recognize the inner child you were when you went through the circumstances and show comfort, support, and love to that little one. Validate that it was a scary and horrible situation and bring love and support to the *little you* that went through it. As if you were a protective parent, your own superhero, or the wiser, better version of yourself and encourage and advise the *young you* so that *young you* can let it go and move on.

Little You

When children experience hurtful or abusive circumstances early in their lives, it is common for them to carry guilt about the abusive situation. This may be true for you. Even though it was someone else's choice to be hurtful to you, you may still think somehow it was your fault or you did something wrong to cause what happened to you.

Please know that it was not your fault! You were just a child. There is nothing you could have possibly done as a child to cause someone else to make bad choices and hurt you. Give that guilt back to the person who deserves it: the person who hurt you, not you. It is not your guilt to carry. Then find the compassion in your heart to forgive them. Not just for them. But mainly for you. If that person is no longer here, forgive them anyway. Then forgive yourself for not knowing it wasn't your fault.

Why We Forgive

Forgiveness allows you to move on. Forgiveness sets you free. Forgiveness gives you closure so you can move forward as a stronger person. Forgiveness clears out negative influences and those rickety old skeletons in the closet so you can create the person you are meant to be and find your true purpose. The older, wiser, and better version of you can help your younger self find freedom and redemption in forgiveness so that you can be at peace.

I used this method myself when I needed to move past some hurtful experiences that surfaced when my husband and I went through our divorce. This is why I love meditation so much. By connecting with my younger self through meditation, I was able to move past obstacles that were subconsciously holding me back. It took some hard work and a lot of forgiveness to get me moving forward again, but eventually, I did. Even now when I feel blocked or unable to move forward with something, I take inventory to discover where unresolved issues in my past may be holding me back. Then I know what to do. It may be something that only happened five or ten years ago, but I still use my older, wiser self to help my younger, less experienced me move through it.

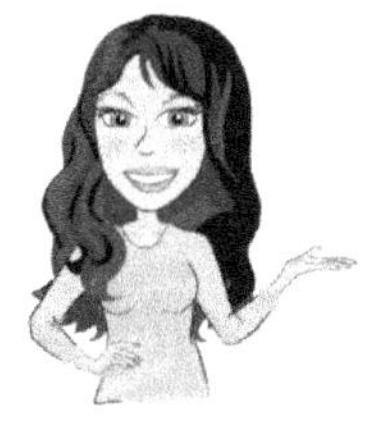

Thinning the Herd

They say nothing in life worth having comes easy and that is no lie. You want a good life? You have to work at it. You want success? You have to be willing to put in the hard work to be successful. You want to find happiness and peace in your life? You have to be real, show up as the person you want to be, and work hard at becoming that person. No one is going to hand a healthy and happy life over to you. They are not going to eat healthily for you or go to the gym and work out for you. They are not going to knock on your door or DoorDash® it to you.

Not one other person is going to complete you! It is not their job, and it is ridiculous and selfish to put that expectation on another person. Their job is to attend to their own journey. If you show up on your journey as the real person you are meant to be, you will not need someone else to complete you. You will realize the only one who can complete you is *you!* The things you were meant to have and the people who were meant to be in your life will be there for you. The things and people who were not meant to be there will fall off to the side because they were not meant to be there!

My grandmother once told me that just because someone is a part of your life at one point or another doesn't mean they are meant to stay in your life forever. This is so true. I remember friends and romantic relationships that contributed positively to my life, and I cherish those. Then there were those that became part of the thinning process. Those people did me a favor by helping me identify the types of people I wanted to surround myself with and those that needed to go. You have to know what you *don't* want in order to know what you *do* want in this life. Thinning the herd is part of that experience.

I have "broken up" with many people in my life that simply did not serve me well. I interact with a core group of people who I am very close to. They love me and encourage the best in me and I in them. There are also people who are positive influences in my life outside of my core group that inspire me and entertain me. All these people are positive influences, and I feed off their positive energy.

Notice I did not mention people who are hurtful, negative, or suck the life out me. That is because I do not let people like that in my personal space. I have worked very hard to create a healthy, happy, and peaceful environment for myself and my family. Don't get me wrong. There are members of my family who have an excuse for everything. Every bad choice they made was someone else's fault. I simply dreaded having conversations with them because it was always the same negative conversation. Years later, nothing changed in their life, so I choose not to interact with them regularly. I love them. I want the best for them, and I wish the best for them in their journey. But I learned the hard way that they have to want the best for themselves in their own journey. Being around negative, hurtful people in no way will help me get where I need to be in my life. If they are meant to be in my life again, it will be when they are ready to make the changes necessary to improve their life. Understand this… you have the right to choose who you want to include on your journey, so choose wisely.

Love and Loss

I have experienced love and loss just like you have. I have suffered rejection just like you have. I have suffered abusive situations just like many of you. I have been hurt deeply and I thought I would never recover from the pain. I have made some really stupid choices and created a few full-on crap storms, and I've had to really humble myself in order to clean them up. I have reinvented myself over and over and shed my skin to the newer, better version of myself many times. Each time I learned more and more about myself and who I am meant to be.

It is not easy to define your life's purpose. Soul search my dear friend! Dig deep down and do not be afraid to shovel through all the crap you have buried. Be courageous and set free the amazing person you were meant to be. Through your courage you will recognize the lessons you were meant to learn. You will find the blessings in the BS that caused you hurt, embarrassment, or distrust. You will find a powerful person who was just waiting for you to release them and let them come to the surface. Be bold, own your crap, then clean that garbage up so you have credibility in this world. When you do this, others will not only respect you, but they will also be inspired by you.

Being a servant does not mean waiting on people hand and foot like I did at Thanksgiving dinner with my grandmother. It means being present to use the gifts and talents you were born with to be a blessing in other people's lives. It means being there when someone needs help and selflessly giving of yourself and your resources, if you have them, to help people who are less fortunate or may be going through difficult times in their journey.

Making it Personal

Once again, take a few moments in a quiet place to write down your thoughts about finding your purpose. What were your natural interests or skills as a child? Do they still inspire you today?

For example, in high school, I seemed to be a natural leader. Without even thinking about it, I managed to influence the other girls; what they wore, getting their ears pierced, doing their makeup. I did use these skills in my early career in the fashion industry, but it was the leadership skills that gave me my purpose. So, think back. What were your interests early in life? What and who inspired you? Did something happen to steer you off that track?

JOURNAL

List what you believe are your best qualities right now. If you have a hard time doing this, ask your best friend or a family member what your top ten qualities are, and write them down. You may find a purpose hiding in there.

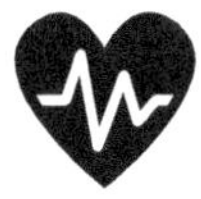

"Forget your perfect offering. There is a crack in everything. That's how the light gets in."
~ Leonard Cohen, Anthem

As I lay in bed, pillows propped behind me to keep somewhat elevated, I felt miserable. A burning sensation crept up my throat while thick mucus dripped down. I had been in bed for a week, struggling to take a deep breath without coughing up a lung. I was overcome with concern that being sick in bed was going to cost me my job. At that time, I held an executive role with the number one fashion house in the world. I believed continuing to work even when I wasn't feeling well demonstrated a strong work ethic. I had so far never missed a day. Being sick just wasn't an option for me. But this time was different.

Truth be told, I hadn't felt well for months. My job was extremely demanding, suited only for someone who could devote 150% to work. Balancing job and family had my stress level spiking off the charts. Add to that my recent divorce and learning how to navigate being single again. This was not one of my finest hours. I was barely keeping it together. Something had to give.

I grabbed my cell phone off my nightstand, called my doctor, and set up an appointment for the following morning. I don't remember the drive to the doctor's office. My head was hopelessly congested, and my lungs were on fire. I had been struggling with a congested cough for almost three months. I kept putting off seeing the doctor about it, simply because I was afraid to take a day off work. (Sound familiar?) My work involved traveling all over the country as an Education Executive. It was extremely difficult to find someone qualified to fill in for me to teach my seminars. If we had to cancel a seminar, it would cost the company a fortune, and I did not want to suffer the consequences of that.

Previous rounds of antibiotics my doctor had prescribed within the last few months had done nothing to improve my condition. During this visit, he decided to do some extensive blood testing in hopes of finding a clue as to why I wasn't getting better. Then he sent me off for more X- rays.

I felt like absolute crap walking down the hall with the x-ray technician, not paying any attention to one word she said as she walked next to me. I was too preoccupied with pushing myself to put one foot in front of the other without falling on my face. After my x-ray, I did my duty and gave what seemed to be half the blood in my body to a nurse, then felt enormous relief to be able to go home and rest while the doctor waited for the results.

He had ordered the tests *stat*, so I was not surprised when he called me a few hours later, requesting I come back in. The drive back to his office was a blur, but I do remember the sobering conversation he had with me when he came in to talk.

A Brick in The Face

"We need to have a serious conversation, Christen." He definitely had my attention now. And what he had to say next hit me like a brick in the face.

"You are prediabetic, your blood pressure is higher than ever before, you have a lung infection that I believe is viral, but I am not sure of the cause. Your immune system has crashed. Your stress level is off the charts, and as I have told you before, stress will take a toll on you if you don't learn to control it. You have gained 40 pounds in the last year which contributes to your chronic acid reflux and prediabetic numbers." Then he looked me in the eye and delivered the final blow. "Christen, you are not going to be here to raise your kids unless make some major changes. Now."

What? That can't be right, can it? I blinked at him in disbelief. I'm a hard charging executive, able to manage a demanding career, a family, a private life, my health, and leap tall buildings in a single bound, right? Apparently not.

He went on again, "I am going to give you six prescriptions. One is a steroid for your lungs, one is for your blood pressure, one for diabetes, one is an antiviral, and one for your acid reflux. Then I am putting you on Lexapro to help with the stress. Most women your age are on Lexapro for stress related to menopause and with your lifestyle, you need stress relief.

Two of these you will only need for a short time, but the other four (for blood pressure, diabetes, acid reflux, and stress) you will need to take from now on."

Seriously? Six Prescriptions!

I sat there stunned as he pushed six pieces of paper into my hands with the information needed to fill my prescriptions. He said he would call the prescriptions in to the pharmacy closest to my house. He then bid me farewell and was on his way to deliver news to the next patient waiting for their diagnosis and most likely a fist full of prescriptions.

Understand this; doctors are not Gods. They are simply trained to identify and treat symptoms. They do not cure diseases. They are also trained through formal schooling and the pharmaceutical companies to treat symptoms with prescription medications. Let me say that again. Their jobs are to identify and treat symptoms of possible diseases. Specialists are trained to diagnose and perform medical treatments in specific areas of their expertise. An example would be a Cardiologist who treats heart conditions. Surgeons can only cure disease if they are able to remove the disease or fix what may be broken through surgical procedures. Ask your doctor if his job is to cure your disease. If he or she is honest, they will say no.

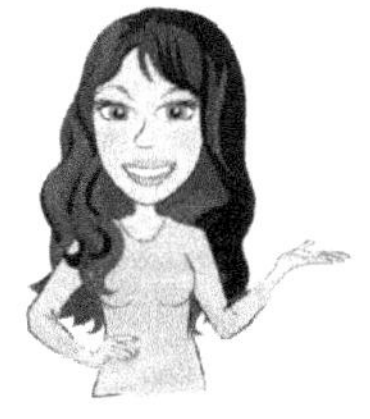

My Come-to-Jesus Moment

I left his office, dragged myself back to my car, and sat in the parking garage for two hours, crying. How had I got myself into this horrific situation? I was so pissed off; first at myself for letting the problems go untreated for so long, then at the doctor. I had been seeing him for years and he just now handed me a fist full of prescriptions (a few of which were unnecessary) instead of discussing possible lifestyle changes that could treat the cause, not just the symptoms. My doctor wasn't there to encourage me to live a healthier lifestyle. If he did, he would soon be out of a job. Instead, I got a five-minute diagnosis, well wishes, and a handful of prescription drugs. Needless to say, he is no longer my doctor.

Sitting there alone in my car, I realized concerns about losing my job were no longer a priority to me. All the hard work and commitment to my company didn't even hit my radar anymore. All I knew was I needed to save my life, and there was no way in hell I was going to take six prescription medications to do that. I most certainly had no intention of filling even one of them! I did have the education about nutrition that could have turned my situation around, and I had ignored it. And that was on me.

As I drove home my anger spiked, fueling an adrenaline rush. I knew what I had to do. I hurried into my house and pulled out several garbage bags from underneath the sink. With heated tears and snot smeared over my face, I started cleaning out my fridge, as colorful words came flying out of my mouth, all aimed at myself for being a dumb ass and putting myself into this situation. When every shelf and drawer in the refrigerator was empty, I moved on to the cupboards. I threw away every bit of junk food and processed crap, and even my favorite chili mac dip. (How many times had chili mac dip comforted me during stressful late-night dates with my computer when I stressed out over getting reports in on time for work? Too many to count.) The dip had to go.

I was amazed at how much junk food I had accumulated. As I slammed box-after-box of crap food out of my cupboards and into the garbage bags, it suddenly hit me. I stopped what I was doing and went back through all the bags I'd loaded from the refrigerator. I did not have one fruit or vegetable in that fridge! Not one. Fifteen years of nutritional education and experience and I was eating nothing but crap food. Even though I had a background in nutrition, the ugly truth was I had allowed myself to fall into the same trap as many of my past clients. The only difference between them and me was I *knew* better. Up until the last two years, I had been coaching clients in nutrition while working in my executive role. Eventually I had to make a choice, so I paused my nutritional business and focused on my commitment to the job that was actually sucking the life out of me.

Owning my S**t

I was 40 pounds overweight, my numbers were the worst they had ever been, and all because I was eating crap food. I was no longer working out even though I knew that behavior would destroy my health. I had allowed my career to take control of my life, meanwhile everything inside of me was falling apart. Literally! I was on a plane and in a different state and hotel five days out of the week. For some reason I had myself convinced that I was immune to all the scary medical conditions associated with poor nutrition because I had a background in nutrition. What an idiot! A background in nutrition did not grant me a get-out-of-jail-free card.

I had to face the fact that I had done this to myself. I had fallen down the same rabbit hole my clients used to come to me to help them out of.

I could blame my job, traveling, stress, my kids, my ex, and my dog for that matter, but the bottom line was, I was the one who put the crap food in my body, and I was the one who allowed poor lifestyle choices to override wisdom. Most importantly, I had let poor lifestyle choices override the necessity to love and care for myself.

No one put a gun to my head and said "Eat that chili mac dip at 11 p.m. with a big bag of tortilla chips. Now, wash it down with a liter of Coke Zero! Do it now or I will blow your head off!" I did it. I ate every chip in that bag and scraped every bite of chili mac dip out of the bowl and shoved it into my mouth.

I made the choice to order pasta rather than a salad for dinner or eggs benedict instead of fruit for breakfast; or eat my favorite chips for a snack instead of nuts or vegetables and hummus. I gave in to the hype and came up with every excuse to justify my poor nutritional choices.

If you think having a nutritional certification makes me a flawless person who doesn't suffer the same temptations and life circumstances as any other working person with an incredibly busy schedule, you are wrong. I have my own set of flaws. In my perfect world, I would love to shove my face into a giant pan of tiramisu and never come up for air. I am Italian and tiramisu has been my favorite dessert since I can remember. I am more like you than you can imagine.

Cleaning Up My Mess

Here is the humbling, embarrassing part. To clean up my "mess," I had to put myself back on my own nutritional program that I had designed for my clients. I literally printed it out and took that flipping program to the grocery store and spent two hours at Whole Foods Market® going through every step I trained my clients to do. I put myself back on my program and followed the same instructions as my clients, including journaling and taking my glucose and blood pressure every morning.

The next day I had to make one of the most difficult choices of my life. I called the Human Resources director at my company and told her I would have to resign from my full-time role. I assumed a part-time role, took a huge pay cut, and gave up a corporate position that most people would die for. Bye-bye big paycheck! Bye-bye high status, jet-setting job!

I needed to find my purpose again. I needed to love myself again. I needed to fix what I had broken. I knew that no one but me was responsible for the choices that had led me to this point in my life, and only I could get myself out of this. That shiny perfect image I presented to the public was a sham. I was broken, and I was the only one who could fix me.

My next adventure was about to begin. It was time to go back to school. I was determined to update my nutritional certificates and once again, reinvent myself.

Learning to Love REAL Food Again

I can't lie, the biggest challenge for me was learning to love the taste of real food again. There were times in my adult life after originally becoming a nutritionist that I fell in love with fruits and vegetables. I especially loved the natural taste of them without sauces, dips, or dressing. (I must have been a rabbit in my past life.) Now it was time to re-program myself and fall in love with the taste of whole foods again.

This is one of the reasons I set up my program to include nothing but plant-based, whole-food nutrition for the first three months. When you are used to eating foods high in saturated fats and sugar, it takes a little time to adjust your palette to eating *clean* food. You must program yourself to love these foods. It is not easy for some people. Others transition with ease like I did. (Maybe they were rabbits in their past lives, too!) All I know is, your body will adapt quickly if you are diligent.

The first step in cleaning up my mess was to start eating every fruit and vegetable I knew would heal my digestive tract quickly. I started with a 16-hour fast and only ate within an 8-hour time frame. I still averaged between 1500 to 1800 calories, but they were healthy, nutrient-dense calories. Foods that loved my body.

My body loved the nutrients I was feeding it, and within one week the lung infection was gone. I did not fill even one of those prescriptions. Keep in mind I was not a full-blown diabetic although my fasting glucose was 135, and my blood pressure was 136 over 75. My normal glucose was in the 85-90 range and my normal blood pressure was 91 over 60. I had always had low blood pressure so 136 was considered high for me. Had I allowed myself to continue eating crap foods, the prescriptions would have become necessary.

A New Adventure

It took three months to lose the 40 extra pounds. I started meditating immediately the day I got home from the doctor. I woke up earlier in the morning if I had to, just to start my day off with the right mental clarity that meditation will almost always provide.

I did weight loss meditations at night while I slept. My body purged itself of the destructive toxins I had been putting into it. The cravings for crap foods soon went away, and I started craving the foods my body needed to heal itself. I no longer craved chili mac dip in times of stress or emotional breakdowns.

I went to the gym and hired the best-looking personal trainer in the place (as I am a visual learner). Having a hottie standing over you while you are busting your ass is great motivation! Could I have trained myself? Yes, however, my trainer was hot, and he held me accountable and that was all the motivation I needed. I had no excuse to not work out. If I tried to cancel on him, he knew how to make me feel guilty enough to talk me out of it.

I found a doctor who was more open-minded when it came to nutrition. I had all of my records transferred to her. I followed-up with her at the end of my three-month journey. My Body Mass Index (weight-to-height ratio) was back in the normal range. My blood pressure was back down to 95 over 65.

Dr. G was impressed. She ordered another blood test and a few days later called me to go over the results. She was more than amazed with what she saw. The numbers were so different, she told me, she actually called the lab to see if there was a possible mix up with another patient. This call was one of the most rewarding calls I had ever received. It went something like this:

"Hi Christen, this is doctor G. I have your blood test results and I wanted to personally call you to discuss them."

My heart started pounding a little hard at that moment. Before she could say another word, I blurted out, "They're better, right?"

She laughed and continued "Better is an under-statement! Your glucose is down to 90, and your cholesterol is back in the normal range. If I didn't know better, I would think I was looking at the results of a healthy 35-year-old woman. Everything looks great!"

I was 49 at that time so that comment really boosted my confidence. My eyes filled with happy tears. "Thank you, thank you, thank you!" I yelled into the phone, unable to control myself.

"I'm not sure what you did," she went on, "but whatever it is, keep doing it. I am very proud of you!" We ended the call on that note. Now the only time she calls me is to tell me to get my butt in for my annual checkups.

Back To School I Go

Back in school, I dove headfirst into my studies. I decided this time I was going to go a different direction with nutrition and focus on clients who were sick from lifestyle diseases, like I had been. I studied the human body and the functions of all the organs. I dug deeply into studies of the digestive system and how all these lifestyle medical conditions are linked to the digestive tract. I did massive amounts of research on leaky gut syndrome and how it is linked to most lifestyle diseases.

After years and years of research as a nutritionist, the biggest *Ah-Ha* moment came when I stepped back and looked at the big picture. Almost every lifestyle disease is linked to poor nutrition.

When people think of nutrition, they associate it with weight loss. Ask the 45 million Americans who go on a diet every year and spend about $33 billion on weight loss products (according to Boston Medical Center). Eighty percent of people who lose weight on fad diets will not maintain the weight loss for even a year (according to Scientific American). Why is this? Because diets are not sustainable. The mind set going in is that they only have to eat "healthy" until they lose some weight and then they go back to eating the Standard American Diet.

What is the Standard American Diet?

The Office of Disease Prevention and Health Promotion defines the Standard American Diet as a modern dietary pattern afflicting American adults and children across the United States with long-term, damaging health consequences.

By definition, the Standard American Diet consists of ultra-processed foods, added sugar, fat, and sodium. Consumption of fruits, vegetables, whole grains, legumes, and lean protein is greatly lacking in this diet.

People also think of fruits and vegetables as "diet" food. The reality is that fruits and vegetables came way before the Standard American Diet. It wasn't that long ago that fruits and vegetables were the foods of choice, with meat only being occasional. This was until the Food Industry started pushing junk food and fast food, and the agricultural business started pushing meat three meals a day! This is why, according to the CDC, our obesity rate has doubled in the past five years.

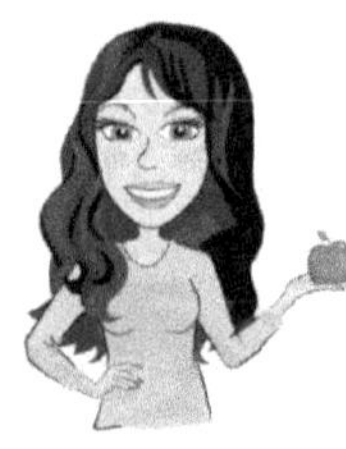

Fruits, vegetables, whole grains, legumes, and lean protein are the very foods we need to heal what's making us sick.

What Is the Answer?

I cannot count the multitude of books I have read and the vast amount of research I have done to find the answer. Over the years I myself have tried all kinds of fad diets in search of the right nutritional program. (Billions of people have tried at least one diet or more.) What works best?

The first, most important and obvious answer is to stop eating foods that are killing you.

Okay, that sounds easy right? If it were only that simple. What we are dealing with is an eating culture, and food choices are a big part of that culture because so many things contribute to why we eat the foods we eat.

Why are 74.6 % of Americans overweight and in the obese categories? I will break it down for you. See if any of this relates to you.

- Americans live by very busy schedules, so food must be easily accessible.

- Americans have become obsessed with electronics and screen time, so they are becoming less active and burning fewer calories.

- In the United States, at least 65% of the Standard American Diet consists of highly processed foods that contain no nutritional value, according to the CDC, so most of the food Americans consume are empty calories, meaning fat calories.

- The American Institute of Stress states that as of 2022, 77% of Americans report experiencing stress that affects their physical health, and 7 % claim stress has impacted their mental health (emotional eating).

- Clinical research shows that 75.7% of Americans in the overweight and obese categories experience "emotional" or "stress eating".

- National Center for Health Statistics from the CDC states that 80% of Americans eat at a fast-food restaurant at least 1-3 times a week.

- According to the CDC, 33% of children and adolescents eat fast food daily.

- According to Fast Food Facts.org, extensive exposure to unhealthy food advertising and marketing increases people's preference to purchase, request, and consume nutritionally poor food products.

- Burgers, pizza, and sandwiches are among the most consumed foods in America.

- Fast food restaurants such as Subway, McDonalds, Dominos, and Burger King spend over 10 million dollars in advertising a year in the United States alone.

- According to the National Institute of Health, food companies use larger portion sizes as selling points. Fast food companies promote larger items and portions sizes to promote sales such as the Double Gulp, and McDonalds Super-Size Meals).

- Consumers are taking in 3 to 4 times the serving sizes and calories recommended per meal.

My clients, and my dad and I regained our health through plant-based, whole-food nutrition. By eating nutrient-dense foods, your body will go into construction mode and start healing itself. Your inflammatory response will be low, and your organs and cells will reset and start doing what they are meant to do.

Think of your digestive system like a factory. It is the most important system in your body because everything depends on it. It needs to function well to keep your body healthy and reach a state of homeostasis or balance. Every cell in your body is fed through your digestive system. Almost everything that enters the blood stream enters through the digestive system. Seventy percent of your immune system is housed in your digestive system so putting crap food in your body means you are feeding every cell and organ in your body, including your brain, so called "food" that is foreign and hostile to its health. Your body does not know what to do with it because it cannot pull any nutrients from the "food" you are putting in it.

The food you eat can either keep your body functioning at it optimum, feeding you energy and giving your cells and organs what the need to keep doing their job well or you can feed your body the typical BS that the Standard American Diet considers food, and you can watch and feel your body fall apart.

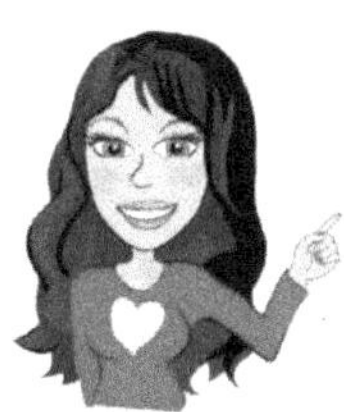

Let me explain something most people miss when it comes to losing weight and most importantly, taking back your health: It is critical that the food you eat be as NUTRIENT DENSE as possible. The more nutrients the better.

My clients will often call me when they are grocery shopping to ask me if they can have "health foods" such as plant-based meat substitutes, dairy free yogurt, or power bars. I have to tell them over and over that just because a food is not necessarily *bad* for you, it doesn't mean it is *good* for you. Is the food you are buying chock full of the nutrients your body needs to heal?

Plant-based meats; dairy free cheeses, yogurts, butters, and power bars are all processed foods. They can and often do have additives, sugars, and saturated and trans fats as well as gluten which causes chronic inflammation. These foods are not going to heal your gut.

Throughout the rest of this book, I go into detail about what nutrient-dense foods to eat that will greatly benefit you and help you take back your health.

TURN YOUR HEART AROUND

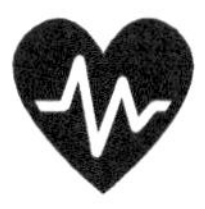

"Everyone has a right to know what is going on inside their body!"

~ Christen Kaplan

We've all heard the phrase "You are what you eat!" Obviously, this does not mean if you eat a piece of pizza, you turn into a slice. Here's what it really means:

Nutritional Foods = Good Health

Standard American Diet (SAD) = Poor Health.

It may surprise you to know that the CDC says the number one cause of premature death in the United States is directly related the Standard American Diet. Unfortunately, I know this all too well. My entire immediate family has suffered devasting consequences due to the SAD diet. (Ironic isn't it, the SAD diet is sad and has the work "die" in it!)

So how do we fix this? In this chapter I am going to leave out the medical jargon and get down to the *nitty gritty* on how eating the right nutrient-dense foods can put you on the path to take back your health.

Following this path isn't easy, but it's simple. You do not have to count calories or weigh your food every day (or yourself for that matter). You simply eat the right food at the right time. It will be difficult in the beginning to part with foods you have become addicted to. You will have to learn a completely new way of eating that at first won't seem as satisfying. It will take a little time to transition into appreciating real foods that will heal your body. It will be important to stand strong and know that eating nutrient-dense food is a major expression of self-love. Your body, in return, will love you for it!

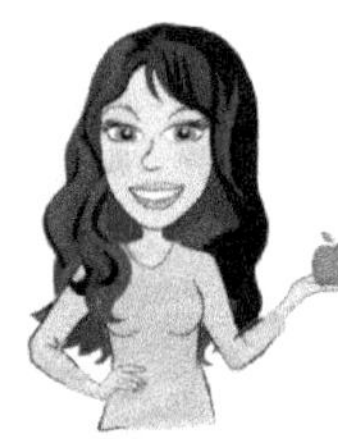

TIMING IS EVERYTHING. *In his books, "The Obesity Code," and "The Diabetic Code", Dr. Jason Fung says that maintaining glucose and insulin balance requires at least a 12-hr fasting period.*

A note on intermittent fasting: An easy way to manage is to not eat anything after 6 p.m. and then not before 6 a.m. (or no less than 4 hours before going to sleep). I like to do a 14-hour fast (nothing to eat between 6 p.m. and 8 a.m.).

When I first transitioned back to eating healthy, I had to change my mind set to eating to live, not living to eat. It did not take long for me to fall in love with the foods that healed my body. When you learn to appreciate why you are eating nutrient-dense foods and what those foods are doing for the organs and systems inside you, it is so much easier.

Here's a great example. I have never been a big fan of broccoli. However, broccoli is a major super food, and one of the healthiest foods you can put in your body. Broccoli is good for heart health, contains cancer protective properties, supports the immune system, reduces inflammation, and improves blood sugar. That is a lot of power packed in one little green vegetable. So, knowing that eating broccoli has so many important benefits, I chose to learn to love it.

This is no joke… I used to cut up my broccoli, put it in a bowl, and then I would verbally thank the broccoli for what it was about to do for my body, and I would eat it. My entire attitude changed about broccoli when I realized what a powerhouse this vegetable was. It took some time and now I crave it. I will take eating broccoli over popping pills any day!

We encourage our clients to be advocates for themselves. Read the printed information that comes with your prescription. Ask questions. You have a right to know why your doctor just prescribed you medication. You have a right to know the side effects of these medications. Why is this important? Because the fourth leading cause of death in the United States is linked to drug interactions. Do not just assume that because your doctor prescribed medication to you that it is your only option.

My sister and I educate and coach a lot of sick and morbidly obese people. It is extremely disturbing to learn how many prescription medications our clients have been given. Ninety-nine percent of them do not know what all of them are for. They just take whatever is prescribed and never question their doctor.

When the doctor handed me six different medications, I researched the possible interactions of these and learned two of the drugs he had prescribed were not meant to be taken together! Had I taken these drugs the way he prescribed, I could have been in serious trouble.

Not too long ago, I was having a conversation with one of my clients' doctors regarding the several medications they had been prescribed. I explained that my client was confused about why he was taking so many medications. When I asked the doctor if he'd explained the reasons for the prescriptions and he said: "My patients don't need detailed information. Most wouldn't understand it even if I had time to explain it."

WTF! (What the fart!) Are you freaking kidding me? This doctor thought so little of his patients that he didn't think they were intelligent enough to understand a basic explanation about what was going on in their own body! What is worse, he assumed they didn't care!

Let's step back and look at that for a moment. There is a legal responsibility to inform patients about their prescription drugs. The pharmaceutical companies are required to issue paperwork about the use and drug interactions of each prescription you take home from the pharmacy. It is the responsibility of the patient to read that documentation to be informed. In some cases, the patient must sign a document at the pharmacy stating they have been informed about the drug and understand how to take it, which lets the pharmacist off the hook.

As I said earlier, doctors are trained to identify disease and treat symptoms. They prescribe drugs to treat those symptoms and leave it to the pharmacist (and the drug manufacturer's lawyers) to inform the patient about the use and side effects of the drug.

They are not currently trained in viable, nutritional alternatives (although, thankfully, this is about to change).

They are not currently *required* to spend time explaining what isn't in their specialty. The time is coming, however. Our national healthcare system is now focusing heavily on preventive medicine. Amen to that! While helping our patients discover the best treatments for lifestyle disease isn't yet a legal responsibility, with the vast majority of Americans suffering the effects of the SAD diet, it is certainly a moral responsibility. A doctor who is truly looking out for your health will point you in the right direction. But the reality is, you must be your own advocate.

You Must Be Your Own Advocate

You not only have a *right* to know what you're putting into your body, self-love demands that you become your own advocate in this regard. Do not let doctors pile on medications like my doctor did.

Don't get me wrong, I'm not advising you to ignore your doctor's orders for prescriptions. What I'm telling you is do not just blindly take what is prescribed without doing your homework. It is up to you to make sure the medication prescribed is absolutely necessary. We're talking about your quality of life here.

In this chapter, I will educate you in the clearest language possible, so you understand you have a choice. All you need is the information necessary to choose for yourself what treatment plans will work best for you. Be an advocate for yourself! Question everything.

A New Approach

First of all, I want you to know we're in this together. We are going to take a different approach to understanding nutrition, health, and your body. By the time you get to the end of this chapter, you will know exactly what you should be putting into your body and why.

You have heard the saying "Feed a man a fish, he eats for a day. Teach a man to fish, he eats for life." That is the approach my sister and I fully believe is the best way for you to learn to take back your health.

Let's shift to a different mindset than what you are used to. We're not going to think of this part of your journey from a weight loss perspective. We're going to focus on your health as a priority. We are going to view your transformation from the inside out.

I promise you: The weight will naturally fall off your body as you love and feed it the right foods. If you eat the way I explain in this book you will have great, long-lasting success. But let's be clear, we are not talking about "diet." We are talking about lifestyle change.

As I educate you in a way that you can understand and appreciate, you will come to love and welcome this change in your life.

First, though, I want to share a story about my sister and how she became a nutritionist. This is hilarious and a true story. She literally lost a bet!

My sister and I have always been somewhat competitive, especially since we are only one year apart. Normally, I am the one going to her for her advice, as she was blessed with wisdom much like my grandmother. One day we were talking on the phone, and she was sharing with me that she was not feeling so good. I asked her what was going on.

She said "I have such horrible acid reflux and I can't sleep at night. I have to prop myself up or I feel like I will throw up."

This was concerning as it is most certainly a common symptom linked to an unhealthy digestive system.

I asked her, "How long has this been going on?"

She said "It has been a while, but it is getting worse. It used to be more at night but now I am getting it during the day too."

My sister lived a healthy lifestyle by most people's standards. She has always loved nutrition, but she still enjoyed some foods that were clearly not agreeing with her. So, we made a deal.

I told her, "I can get rid of your acid reflux in two days."

She said, "I am not sure of that, Sis. It's pretty bad. I am eating Tums like candy!"

"I will make a deal with you," I told her. "A wager if you will. If I can get rid of your acid reflux in 48 hours, you must go back to school and get your Holistic Nutrition Certification and come and partner with me. If I can't then you can have anything you want from me."

"I like where this is going," she said. "Anything, huh?"

"Yes, anything!"

She, feeling very confident, agreed. She thought it would be impossible to get rid of acid reflux in 48 hours.

I gave her very clear instructions on how to get rid of her annoying acid reflux. I put her on my program and in the morning of the third day, she called me.

"Sis, I guess I am going back to school! As much as it pains me to admit it, you were right! The acid reflux is gone and for the first time in a long time I slept through the night and went all day with no discomfort at all."

"Whoo Hooo!" I shouted, jumping up and down. "I won! I won!" Then I sent her all the information she needed to enroll in classes.

Now my sister is my business partner and an excellent Nutritionist. She is also the co-author with me of the Take Back Your Health series.

We are really proud of these books as they provide critical information to educate you so you can make the right choices for you and your loved ones. Use these books often as references when you need a refresher or when you are done with them, share them with someone else who can benefit. Pay it forward!

Getting Our Plants On

So far in this book, I have focused on the mind, body, and soul connection. I have also shared my personal experiences and the journey my father took to regain his health. Now I want to share some life changing information to get you started on your own journey to regaining your health and vitality.

Hopefully you have already begun using the tools in this book to clear your mental house and leap over obstacles that have been holding you back. Now we get to focus on your body. This is my favorite discussion because nutrition to me is almost like a religion. I have read hundreds of books on nutrition over the last 20 years and researched every diet you can imagine. I have taken countless classes and seminars and done extensive research on plant-based nutrition, the human body, and the SAD diet. Needless to say, nutrition is my jam!

Years of research clearly show that diets do not work. Clearly, if you are reading this book, you have tried a few and can agree with me. Diets are simply not sustainable. Countless research studies show that less than five % of people on a typical fad diet will have long term success. Why? Because "diets" foster a temporary mindset. "Lose 30 pounds by Summer!"

says the magazine in the checkout stand. And when summer's over, it's back to your old eating habits.

To maintain long-term success, you must make long-term changes to your eating and lifestyle habits. You must completely change your relationship with food. Food can no longer be a crutch or a self-soothing tool.

As you learned earlier, food isn't just something you put in your mouth for a temporary rush of satisfaction. Food is meant to nourish your body and feed the cells and internal organs what they need to maintain a state of homeostasis (balance). Every cell and organ in your body has a job to do. Proper nutrition helps ensure that the organs and cells have all the tools they need to do their job.

Under Construction

If you are suffering from lifestyle disease, your digestive tract needs to be reconstructed. Literally. So, we are going to put your body "under construction." We are going to rebuild your health from the inside out, starting with your digestive tract.

Think of your cells and organs as little construction workers laboring away in your body, non-stop, 24 hours a day, to keep you healthy and thriving. Then, out of nowhere, a food storm (the SAD diet) hits your construction site (your digestive tract) destroying everything your workers have labored to build.

Multiply the SAD diet by three meals a day and it becomes a tsunami, making it impossible for your construction workers (cells) to get the tools and materials (nutrients) they need to repair the damage. They are literally under attack all day long.

It doesn't take long before your construction site (digestive tract) is reduced to rubble and your workers are left defenseless as they come under attack again and again; three meals a day, day-after-day, with no help in sight.

Now your safety net (immune system) breaks down. Your safety team (immune cells) call in sick and go on strike because of unhealthy work conditions. There are no more healthy construction workers left to clean up the mess, and your health spirals out of control. Your blood pressure and cholesterol elevate, and you are becoming diabetic!

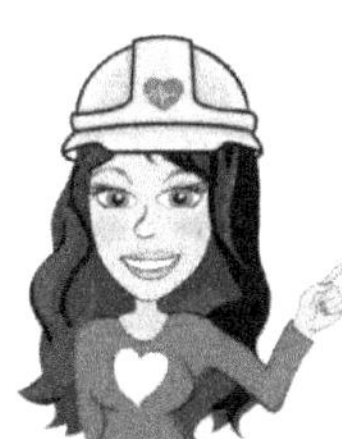

FEAR NOT! *Help is on the way! Superheroes (nutrient dense foods/plant based whole food nutrition) are ready to come to the rescue.*

Calling All Superheroes!

You decide to fight for your health! Yay!!! Help is on the way!

There is a major shift in the weather and all your favorite superheroes (nutrient-dense fruits and vegetables) defeat the SAD diet and begin to rescue your construction workers. The superheroes clean up the mass destruction in your digestive tract caused by the SAD tsunami. Your workers are so happy their construction site is clean, they band together and come back to work.

Your superheroes continue to deliver all the tools your workers need to do their job. Peace and good health are on the horizon! Before you know it, your construction site becomes a strong and beautiful headquarters for the rest of your body as you finally return to a state of homeostasis (balance).

The Digestive Tract is Your Body's Headquarters

It's easy to think of your brain as your body's headquarters, but that's not really the case. The digestive system is your body's headquarters. The digestive system feeds the brain. The digestive system breaks down food into nutrients that can then be absorbed into the blood stream so the body can use these nutrients for energy, growth, and healing.

The digestive system is also responsible for the excretion of waste products. Remember, when I referred to my body as a fine Ferrari? This is where putting the right fuel in your gas tank comes into play. My body was meant to take in nutrient-dense foods as premium fuel. Putting in nutrient-deficient foods will obviously have a negative effect on the way my engine runs. It is like putting peanut butter in your gas tank instead of premium fuel. Your digestive tract was not meant to digest processed junk and foods high in sugars, sodium, and saturated and trans fats. All these foods cause you to not only store fat, but also create chronic inflammation.

If you are suffering from frequent discomfort, GERD, (chronic acid reflux), loose stools or constipation, heartburn, gas, bloating, weight gain, or chronic fatigue, these are warning signs that your digestive system is in a major crisis. If you are having trouble sleeping, this is another red flag. Most serotonin (your body's feel-good hormone) is produced in your gut. When inflammation caused by consuming foods high in sugars, sodium, and saturated and trans fats flood your digestive system, it can cause insomnia or disrupted sleep patterns.

Over the course of this series, my sister and I will explain in layman's terms, each of the major medical conditions associated with poor nutrition, why you or your loved ones have the condition, what is happening to cause the condition, and lastly, how to fix it.

Our nutritional program is successful because we believe education is power. Learning is power, and educating yourself is an expression of Radical Self-Love. So, let's dive in and get started talking about nutrition.

The Pillars of Good Nutrition

"Your health is powerfully determined by how well you live your life."

~ Dr. Dean Ornish, M.D.

By now you know I'm an advocate for Radical Self-Love. How well you love and care for yourself will determine how well you will live your life. The way you eat is one of the most important factors when it comes to living a healthy and vibrant life. Nutrient-dense foods feed the body, mind, and soul well. There is no doubt that when I eat healthy, I feel better in my body, mind, and soul. Plants have a life source to share with you when you consume them. They deliver massive amounts of nutrients, vitamins, minerals, and phytonutrients that feed every cell in your body.

Let's take a look at the food groups that fit into the category of nutrient-dense foods. The following food groups work like powerful superheroes when it comes to cleaning out your digestive system and healing it.

Remember the acid reflux story I told you about my sister? Within a few days of eating the following foods, her acid reflux was gone. This is a common response when you put the proper food in your digestive tract. Right now, if you are sick due to lifestyle disease, are overweight or obese, or have any or many of the frequent discomforts I listed in the previous paragraphs, please pay close attention. Your digestive tract is unhealthy. The following foods will help you repair the damage. You will not starve. I promise you. Most of my clients come back to me and say they cannot eat this much food:

- *Fruits (3 servings a day preferably with breakfast or lunch)*

- **Berries (1 serving. Very high in antioxidants)*

- *Leafy greens (2 servings a day)*

- *Cruciferous Vegetables (1 serving a day)*

- *Other vegetables (2 servings a day)*

- *Whole grains (2 servings a day)*

- *Beans (2 servings a day)*

- *Nuts and seeds (1 serving a day)*

- *Flaxseed (1 serving s day)*

All these foods help heal the digestive tract and lower blood pressure and blood sugar. These foods also quickly and dramatically reduce acid reflux. If you have chronic acid reflux, you want to avoid acidic foods, saturated fats, highly processed foods, and alcohol. The more greens, berries, cruciferous vegetables, and other vegetables, fruits, and whole grains you can put into your body the better. Eating late at night or right before bed will also contribute to acid reflux.

Let's break down the benefits of these foods so you can see how they apply to your medical condition. First, I want to introduce you to two important elements that make fruits and vegetables your superhero foods: **Fiber** and **Antioxidants**. Then we will break down each food group.

FIBER

Cambridge Dictionary defines Fiber as: Noun - A substance in plant foods such as fruits and vegetables, that is not broken down during the digestive process, then travels through the digestive system and helps the contents of the bowels pass easily through the body.

Most people associate fiber with regulating bowel movements, and that is an important benefit, but fiber has several additional and very important benefits, which is why fiber should be a daily part of your nutritional program. Let's take a look at a few of them:

- *Balances cholesterol levels*

- *Helps regulate blood sugar*

- *Helps lower high blood pressure*

- *Improves healthy gut microbiome*

- *Promotes regular bowel movements*

- *Keeps you feeling full longer*

- *Reduces the risk of heart disease*

- *Reduces the risk of type-2 diabetes*

- *Reduces the risk of colorectal cancer*

Fiber is classified in two categories, **soluble** and **insoluble.**

Soluble fiber dissolves in water and can aid in several of the benefits listed above. **Insoluble fiber** promotes the movement of material through the digestive system and aids in regulating healthy bowel movements. There are so many other benefits I can't include them all here, but the following are some of the most beneficial elements.

Foods high in fiber and other nutrients include:

- Avocado - Full of healthy fats, beneficial to heart health, high in vitamin C, potassium, magnesium.

- Artichokes - Rich in nutrients, packed full of Vitamins and minerals, supports heart health, healthy blood pressure, may improve liver health, and improves digestive health.

- Apples - Have over 10,000 phytonutrients, lowers risk of diabetes, heart disease, and cancer, promotes weight loss, and improves gut and brain health.

- Almonds - Good source of vitamin E, high in protein, fiber and healthy fats, and calcium.

- Beans - High in fiber, protein, iron, potassium, zinc, boost heart health, support healthy blood sugar.

- Broccoli - Supports a healthy gut, good for heart health, provides cancer protective compounds, supports the immune system, supports weight loss, and helps regulate blood pressure.

- Brussels sprouts - Excellent source of soluble fiber, high in vitamins and minerals, high in folate, supports a healthy gut, supports heart health, supports the immune system.

- Brown rice – Provides calcium, magnesium, vitamins B1 and B6.

- Bananas – Provides potassium, magnesium, vitamin C and B6.

- Chia seeds - High in nutrients, supports digestive health, can assist in weight loss.

- Chickpea - High in nutrients, proteins, and minerals.

- Carrots - Helps prevent constipation, high in beta carotene, antioxidants, and potassium.

- Lentils - Very high in protein and considered one of the healthiest foods on this earth.

- Kidney beans - High in fiber, protein, great source of iron.

- Quinoa - High in protein and fiber and can be found gluten free.

- Oranges - High in vitamin C, fiber, helps body absorb iron, and boosts immune system.

- Split pea - High in protein, iron, zinc and phosphorus.

- Strawberry - High in antioxidants, magnesium, calcium, folate, potassium, and vitamin K.

- Sweet potato - High in vitamin A, beta carotene, and antioxidants; promotes healthy gut and brain.

- Pears - Excellent source of soluble and insoluble fiber, high in nutrients, anti-inflammatory, protects against cancer, supports heart health, improves blood pressure, helps lower cholesterol.

Obviously, fiber is very important. Processed foods and animal products do not contain the fiber you need to support a healthy digestive tract. Fiber comes only from plants. The SAD diet not only has little to no fiber, but it is also <u>nutrient deficient,</u> meaning most of the SAD diet has no nutritional value at all.

ANTIOXIDANTS

Oxford languages defines Antioxidants as: A substance that is used to counteract the deterioration, and damaging oxidizing agent in a living organism.

I want to scream this from the roof tops! Antioxidants are *soooo* important! Antioxidants are the superheroes that protect the cells, tissue, and organs inside your body. Antioxidants are like a protective dome over your body, inside and out. Fruits and vegetables are high in antioxidants and 100% necessary to heal and protect your body. Animal foods and processed foods that make up the SAD diet do not have antioxidants to protect your body. As a matter of fact, the SAD diet is what is killing our people.

Let's take a look at some of the superheroes high in antioxidants that protect your body, and some of their additional benefits:

- Berries - blackberries, blueberries, strawberries, cranberries, goji berries, are all HIGH in antioxidants, LOW in calories, and HIGH in fiber. Wild blue berries and blackberries top the list. They deliver vitamins A and C, as well as flavonoids (a type of antioxidant).

- Red peppers - Full of carotenoids that can help prevent cancer, also HIGH in fiber and LOW in calories.

- Artichokes - Topping the list for antioxidant power, an excellent source of fiber, and major health benefits associated with this veggie.

- Sweet potatoes - Helps support a healthy immune system, excellent source of fiber, loaded with nutrients.

- Walnuts - Loads of polyphenols (a type of antioxidant), one of healthiest nuts you can eat. Countless nutritional benefits.

- Tomatoes – Great source of potassium, vitamin K, vitamin C, and folate for tissue and cell growth, and lycopene, protects against heart disease and cancer.

- Dark chocolate - 80% cocoa, very high in anti-oxidants, decreases inflammation, reduces risk of heart disease.

- Leafy green vegetables (spinach, kale, arugula, and chard) may be one of the best cancer preventive foods. Aids in healing the digestive system, lowers blood pressure, helps regulate blood sugar, high in fiber, and very high in nutrients.

- Red cabbage - Good source of vitamin K, calcium, magnesium, zinc, and fiber. Supports a healthy digestive system.

- Beans - High in fiber, protect against heart disease, regulates blood pressure and blood sugar. Supports healthy digestive tract.

- Parsley – Rich in vitamin C and K, helps reduce the risk of heart disease, high blood pressure, supports bone health.

- Prunes - Helps digestion, high in fiber, regulate bowel movements, high in vitamins, lowers cholesterol levels, and lower blood pressure.

- Oregano – Anti-bacterial, anti-viral, anti- inflammatory, anti-cancer properties, supports the immune system.

- Turmeric - Anti-inflammatory, supports a healthy heart, anti-cancer, promotes healthy respiratory, digestive tract, liver, and reduces inflammation due to arthritis.

- Plums - Rich in vitamins and minerals, high in potassium and Vitamin C, rich in polyphenols, can reduce the risk of cardiovascular disease.

- Kiwi - Contains serotonin, flavonoids, can improve sleep, lower blood pressure, reduce the risk of heart disease, high blood pressure and stroke.

- Green tea - Fat burning, may improve brain function, may lower the risk of cancer, help reduce type-2 diabetes, and may help prevent heart disease.

- Flaxseed - High in fiber, good for the digestive tract, lower cholesterol levels, rich in omega-3, reduce the risk of osteoporosis.

I could go on and on with the list of foods important for supporting a healthy body. Can your cheeseburger do that? Donuts? Fried foods? The Standard American Diet?

Fruits and Berries

Think of fruits and berries as your antioxidant superheroes using their superpowers to put a protective force field over your body.

In an article on *NutritionFacts.org*, Dr. Michael Greger, M.D., FACLM, states that "plant-based foods have 64 times more antioxidant power than red meat, poultry, fish, dairy, and eggs."

According to the National Center for Biotechnology, an article titled *"Can Meat and Meat-Products Induce Oxidative Stress?"* concluded that meat product consumption has been related to degenerative diseases due to saturated fatty acids and high cholesterol content.

With the majority of Americans suffering from the effects of the SAD diet; fruits, berries, and vegetables have never been more important than they are now as the way to turn peoples' health around. They are an excellent source of vitamins, minerals, fiber, antioxidants, and they can reduce your risk and help reverse the effects of heart disease, high blood pressure, high cholesterol, and type-2 diabetes, many cancers, inflammatory disease, and stroke. They can assist in regulating some of the symptoms of Type 1 diabetes as well.

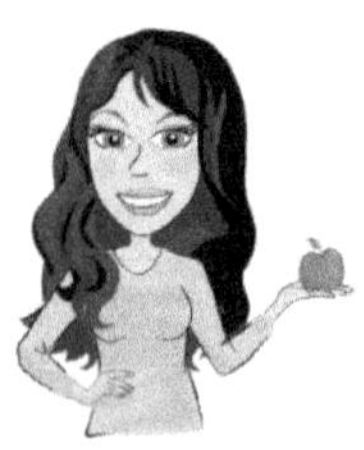

Even with high fruit and berry intake, I recommend my clients take a magnesium supplement to support muscle and bone and help regulate the digestive tract. Taken at night, it can also promote peaceful sleep.

Citrus fruits contain vitamin C, folic acid, potassium, magnesium, and lots of fiber and pectin, all of which help support a healthy immune system.

In the following lists of superhero foods, you will find certain foods with an *. These are Super *Duper* Superhero foods. Try to include as many as you can in your daily food intake.

***Blackberries**	***Raspberries**	**Strawberries**
***Blueberries**	**Cranberries**	***Apples**

*Avocados	*Kiwi	Passion fruits
Bananas	*Lemons	Peaches
Cantaloupe	Limes	*Pears
Clementines	Lychees	Pomegranate
Dates	Mangos	Prunes
Dried figs	Nectarines	*Plums
Grapefruit	*Oranges	Tangerines
Honey dew	Papaya	Watermelon

Leafy Greens

Dark, leafy greens are one of the healthiest foods on the planet. As whole foods go, they offer the most nutrients per calorie. Harvard University researchers promote eating leafy greens as the strongest protection against major chronic diseases including up to a 60% reduction in the risk of both heart attacks and strokes if eaten three servings a day. Leafy greens protect your DNA and are especially important for those at risk for heart disease, stroke, and type-2 diabetes.

The following is a list of your most popular leafy green heroes. Again, those with and * are the highest nutrient value and you should include as many as you can in your daily food intake. (Note: some leafy greens also fit into the cruciferous category.)

*Arugula	Collard green
Beet greens	

Kale (black, green and red)

Sorrel

Mesclun mix

Spinach

Mustard greens

Swiss chard

Turnip greens

Cruciferous Vegetables

Cruciferous vegetables like broccoli and cauliflower can potentially prevent DNA damage and may reduce the spread of metastatic cancer if eaten with an anti-inflammatory diet. Cruciferous veggies can defend against pathogens and pollutants, may help to prevent lymphoma, boost liver detox enzymes, and reduce the risk of prostate and breast cancers. The component responsible for these benefits is an anticancer agent called sulforaphane. Sulforaphane is also responsible for protecting your brain and eyesight, reducing nasal allergy inflammation, and helps manage type-2 diabetes.

Notably, in a 2017 small study published by the "Global Advances in Health and Medicine," and listed the "National Library of Medicine," it was found that the sulforaphane from broccoli sprouts could significantly reduce the behavioral symptoms of Autism Spectrum Disorder, a disease that affects 1 in 68 young people in this country.

Here are your Cruciferous Vegetable heroes. Note: One * means once again they are high value, and two ** means they belong both in the leafy and cruciferous categories.

*Broccoli

*Brussels sprouts

Bok choy

*Cauliflower

Cabbage

**Collard greens

**Kale (black, green, and red)

**Mustard greens

**Turnip greens

Horseradish

Radishes

Watercress

Other Vegetables

Other Vegetables

All vegetables have nutrient value. These are some of the other vegetables that contribute to a healthy body. We can't leave these guys out. Full of nutrients and vitamins and minerals, these veggies all have incredible benefits to your health.

*Artichokes

*Asparagus

*Beets

Bell peppers

Carrots

Corn

Garlic

*Mushrooms

Okra

Onions

*Purple potatoes

Pumpkin

Snap peas

Squash

*Sweet potatoes

Tomatoes

Zucchini

Legumes

Legumes contain a plethora of health benefits that include being high in protein and fiber, assisting with weight loss, and assisting in detoxing and removing body waste. They also fight inflammation and heart disease and help decrease cholesterol. They are high in antioxidants and can help prevent cancer. Beans are naturally low in saturated fat, sodium, and free of cholesterol.

Here is a nice list of your legume heroes (Eat lots of the ones with *):

*Black beans

Black-eyed peas

Butter beans

Chickpeas

English peas

*Great northern beans

Kidney beans

*Lentils

Miso

Navy beans

Pinto beans

*Small red beans

*Split peas

Nuts and Seeds

Nuts make for a quick and delicious snack. The healthiest of these being the walnut. Walnuts are highest in antioxidants and omega 3's in the nut family. Nuts and seeds are also high in protein, fiber and antioxidants. Fun fact: Brazil nuts are known for lowering cholesterol if eaten 2 to 3 times weekly. Be careful though not to eat too much. They also have selenium which in the right amount is really good for you but can be dangerous if you consume too much.

Nuts and Seeds heroes:

*Walnuts

Almonds

*Brazil nuts

Chia Seeds

Cashews (small amounts, higher in fat)

Hazelnuts

Hemp seeds

Macadamia nuts

Pecans

Pistachios

Pumpkin seeds

Sesame seeds

Sunflower seeds

Whole Grains

Whole grains are a necessary and important part of plant-based nutrition. Some fad diets try to minimize the importance of whole grains and even go as far as to recommend you cut them out of your diet completely. I could not disagree more. Whole grains reduce the risk of heart disease, type-2 diabetes, obesity, and stroke. Focus on gluten free and organic when possible. There are so many options.

Is it really whole grain?

Beware! Not everything labeled "whole grain" is the real deal. By law, food companies are allowed to label a package "whole grain" as long as there is any amount listed in the ingredients. Especially bread and crackers. The best way to tell if your bread is a true whole grain is to look at the label. If the amount of carbohydrates divided by fiber comes out to 5 or less. You have a real whole grain product. Here's a shot of a popular whole grain brand that is the real deal.

Nutrition facts	^
1.0 servings per container	
Serving size	1 Slice (45g)
Amount per serving	
Calories	110

% Daily Value*

Total Fat 1.5g	
Saturated Fat 0g	
Trans Fat 0g	
Cholesterol 0mg	
Sodium 170mg	
Total Carbohydrate 22g	
Dietary Fiber 5g	
Sugars 4g	
Protein 6g	
0%	Vitamin A
0%	Vitamin C
2%	Calcium
7%	Iron
	Potassium 100mg

*The % Daily Value (DV) tells you how much a nutrient in a serving of food contributes to a daily diet. 2,000 calories a day is used for general nutrition advice.

Here is a list of popular whole-grain heroes:

Barley

Brown rice

Buckwheat

Millet

Raw organic gluten free oats

Quinoa

Rye

Brown rice pasta

Whole grain pasta

Organic wild rice

Herbs and Spices

While we are at it, I want to list some herbs and spices that have nutritional value and are good for seasoning without high contents of sodium.

Allspice	*Dill*	*Smoked pap-rika*
**Basil*	**Fenugreek*	**Parsley*
Bay leaf	*Garlic*	*Pepper*
Cardamom	**Ginger*	*Peppermint*
Chili powder	*Horseradish*	*Rosemary*
Cilantro	*Lemongrass*	*Saffron*
**Cinnamon*	*Marjoram*	*Sage*
Cloves	*Mustard powder*	*Thyme*
Coriander	*Nutmeg*	**Turmeric*
**Cumin*	**Oregano*	*Vanilla*
Curry pow-der		

I feel like I cannot say this enough. ***"Nothing tastes as good as healthy feels."*** All of the foods, herbs, and spices listed offer incredible benefits to your body, mind, and soul. These foods offer an opportunity to fix the long list of lifestyle disease that have become a major crisis here in America thanks to the Standard American Diet.

The American Food Industry is not Your Friend

The food industry is not interested in making you healthy. There is not enough money in it for them when they can make a lot more money from making you sick. It is no coincidence that two of the biggest money makers in this country are the fast food and meat industries (USD $522 billion combined) and big pharma ($424 billion). Between the two, that is almost a trillion dollars! Is it a surprise that 74.6% of Americans are overweight, obese, and unhealthy?

I will leave you with this thought... When was the last time you saw a TV commercial advertising fruits and vegetables? When was the last time you saw a commercial advertising a healthy lifestyle such as exercising, drinking more water, getting a good night's sleep, eating healthy, or managing stress naturally using natural stress management techniques? Okay... Now, how many fast-food commercials do you see during every show? Processed food commercials like sugary boxed cereals and mac and cheese? Prescription drug commercials? Do you get my point?

Making it Personal

Time to record more in your Journal. Think about your regular grocery list. What foods do you buy every time you go shopping because that's what you always buy? Now look at the list of foods in this chapter. How many of those foods show up on your regular grocery list? Can you add some superfood construction workers to your list? What foods can you swap out completely to stop the destruction of your digestive tract?

JOURNAL

NOTES

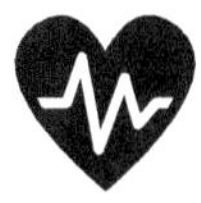

Now that you've bolstered your emotional courage, dumped the baggage that's been holding you back, are beginning to show yourself the Radical Self-Love you deserve, and have begun to include in your daily meals the nutrient-rich foods that can literally turn your heart around, it's time to tackle the physical damage obesity has done to your body. The next books in the "Take Back Your Health!" series hold the key to reclaiming a happy, healthy, rewarding life for you and your loved ones.

Trust that you are wise enough, intelligent enough, and regardless of where you are in your life right now, you have the courage to tackle the changes you need to reclaim your journey and reclaim your health. There is a higher version of yourself waiting for you in your future. You just need to give yourself the tools and nutrient-rich foods you need to break free from the challenges of lifestyle disease.

Do not beat yourself up for letting things get out of hand with your health. With nearly 75% of Americans overweight or obese, you are definitely not alone. It mostly comes down to the fact that you don't know what you don't know. I didn't either until I became a nutritionist. After reading this book, you know a heck of a lot more than you did before you picked it up. My hope is you have already begun to make small changes in your life that can pay big dividends down the road.

The next step is to continue to educate yourself so you can make wise choices for a healthy, fulfilled, future you. The next book in this series builds on what you have learned in *Turn Your Heart Around* as I continue to share with you my family's stories along with the no BS truth about lifestyle diseases and how you can take back your health.

Before You Move On

Before you move on to the next book, I want to formally introduce my sister, Elizabeth (Beth) Inman, co-owner with me and COO of *Love a Wholistic Life, Inc.,* and our sister company, *Integrative Wholistic Diagnostics, Inc.* Her extensive business background with JP Morgan Chase was foundational in preparing her for this dual role.

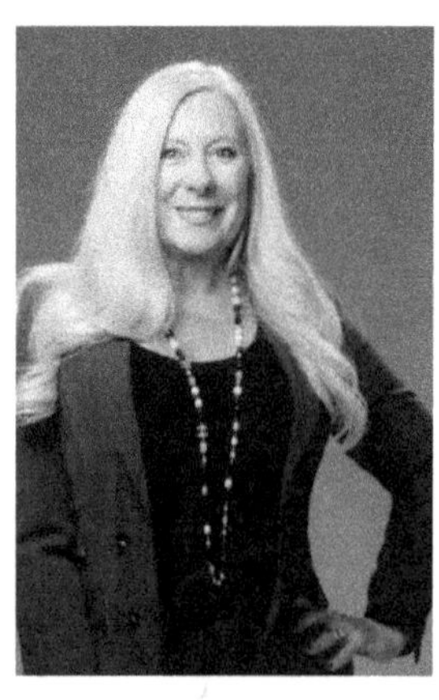

Like me, she is an AFPA Certified Holistic Nutritionist and Weight Counselor. (I told you how that came about back in Chapter 10). She is not only my sister, but also my BFF, my soulmate, and my partner in crime. She is a year older than I am, so she is also my big sister. She ALWAYS has my back. She is one of the wisest women I know, and she is a servant to others like I am. I am the creative one, always off chasing butterflies; she is the one who keeps me on a retractable leash to reel me in when I need to focus (metaphorically speaking).

You will be hearing a lot more from Beth as she is the co-author with me of the next books in the series.

To learn more about our work helping clients overcome the devastation of lifestyle disease, visit our website and follow us on your favorite social media:

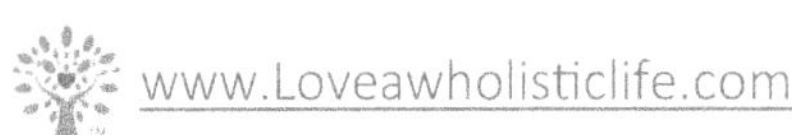 www.Loveawholisticlife.com

christen.kaplanutrition   eliza.bethinman

loveawholisticlife

@christenkaplanutrition   @elizabethinmannutrition

@ChristenLoveAWholisticLife

If you or someone you love is struggling with lifestyle disease, our Take Back Your Health series is custom made to help you understand how lifestyle diseases affect the body and introduce the tools needed to counter the effects and regain control over your health. If you haven't already read Book 1, we invite you to check it out as it delivers a massive dose of experience, compassion, and no BS support to understand and implement the changes necessary to reclaim your health.

BOOK 1 – *Turn Your Heart Around!*

*The Mind, Body, & Soul Connection to Prevent &
Reverse Lifestyle Disease*

BOOK 2 – *Defeat Type 2 Diabetes*

The Kick-Ass Nutrition Guide to Prevent and Overcome Type-2 Diabetes

 A colorful, easy to use 90-day journal to help you stay on track with your take back your health journey.

BOOK 3 –*The Lies Your TV Tells You*

*Breaking Free of the Marketing Traps Promoted by
the Food Industry, Big Pharma, and the Media.
(Coming soon)*

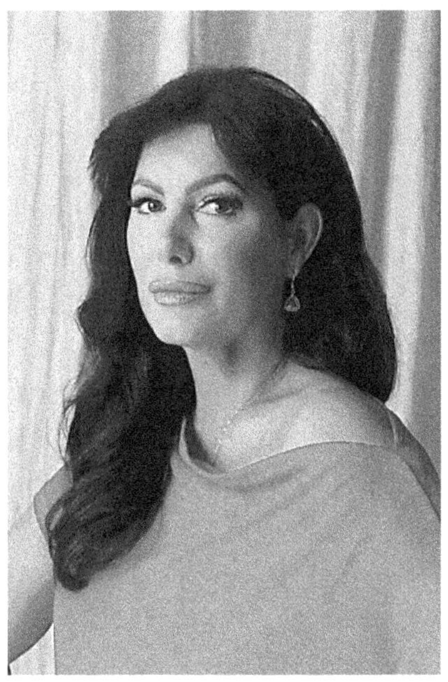

Christen Kaplan is the Co-Owner and CEO of Love a Wholistic Life, Inc. She is an AFPA Certified Holistic Nutritionist and Supplementation and Wellness Expert. She has held certifications as a CPT, Post Rehab Specialist, Level 1 Postural Assessment Specialist and Medical Exercise Specialist.

Christen's corporate experience includes 12 years in the fashion industry where she committed her life to a rigorous executive corporate structure with two of the top fashion houses in the world. It was an amazing experience, but the unbalanced lifestyle came at great personal cost to her and her family. She knew it was time to make some changes and left Corporate America to follow her calling.

Christen and her sister, Elizabeth co-founded Love a Wholistic Life, Inc., with a passion to educate and help people achieve true, lasting health. Like many Americans, Christen's family has suffered loss due to preventable lifestyle diseases. Through this experience, it has become a lifelong mission to help clients restore and maintain their health.

Christen lives in Orange County, CA with her two teenagers and two Labrador retrievers. She also serves as the Program Director for the *Associazione Familia De Mon Rubro Monte* in Monterosso Calabro, Italy where she owns a home and spends three months a year. Christen and her fellow members in the *Associazione* initiate programs and raise funding to ensuring the townspeople live in clean, beautiful, thriving communities.

When she isn't teaching, working with clients or blogging, Christen is perfecting her Italian, snuggling with her dogs, or spending the day painting in her studio. She also loves yoga and video chatting with her sister.

I want to thank my Editor, Katina Drennan for working so closely with me and encour-aging me to write from my heart. Without her this book would not have been possible.

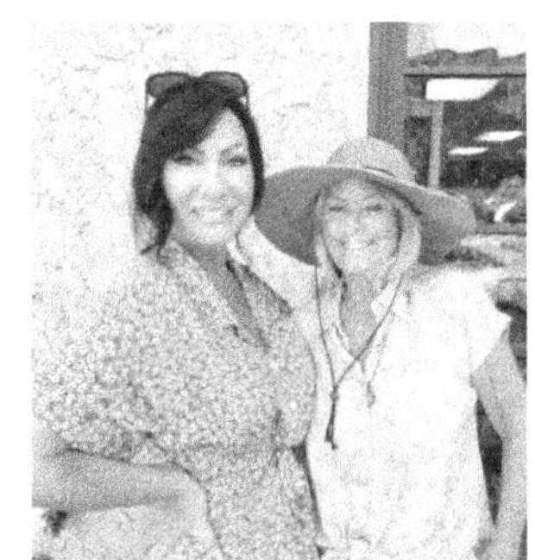

I also want to thank another hero in my life, E. Jeffrey Galloway for all of your love and support. You have always believed in me and have encouraged me to be the best version of myself by leading by example.

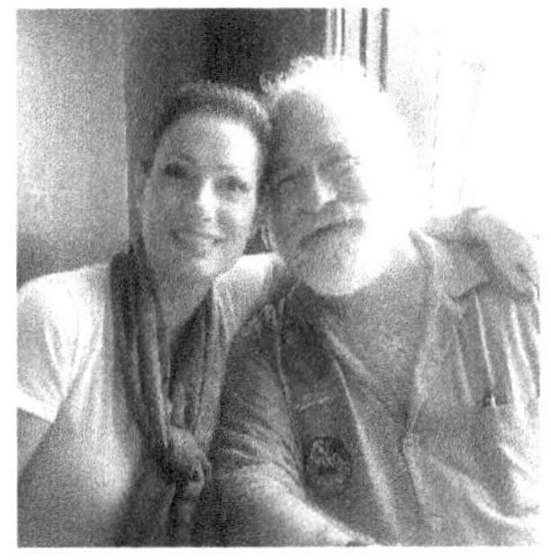

Another big thank you to my soul sister, Stephanie Shahabi. You built in me a fierce and powerful woman by being a beautiful example of that yourself. Thank you for putting a fire under my ass and laughing through hard times with me. You are my inspiration.

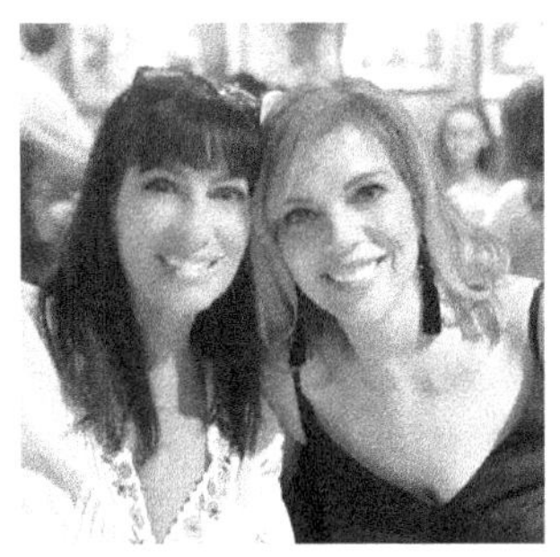

I want to thank my partner, best friend and sister, Elizabeth Inman for keeping me focused, being my voice of reason, and never letting me forget why we do this.

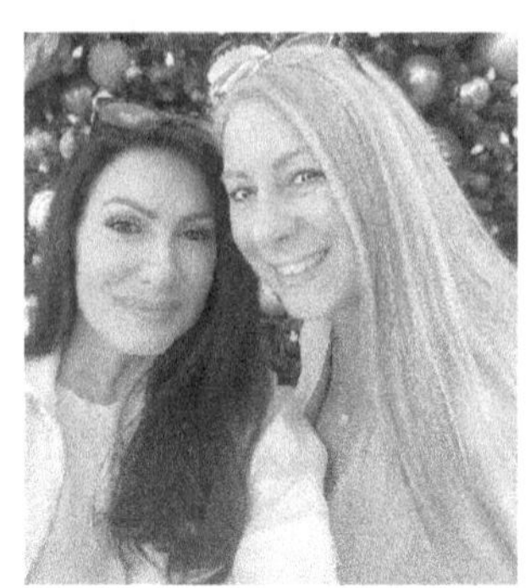

Last but not least, I want to thank my brother, Jason for being my biggest fan. You raise me up through your encouragement and deep love for your sisters. You are an amazing man.

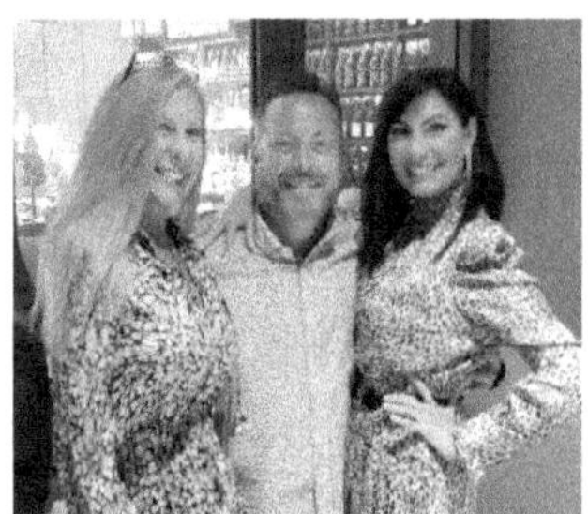

Disclaimer - I do not get paid or receive benefits of any kind for these referrals. These are simply resources that have played a big role in my education and success in both my professional and personal growth.

Nutritional

The following books are excellent references to understanding lifestyle diseases and how to heal the body. Most of these books were written by renowned medical doctors who are experts in the field of medicine and nutrition. Please do your research on each book that appeals to you. Some of these books will take some time to get through and some are easy reads. All are important. I have put an * next to my favorites, but I really love all of them. Throughout this series I will be adding more to this list at the end of each book, but this is a great start.

*How Not To Die, Dr. Michael Greger

*How Not To Diet, Dr. Michael Greger

The longevity Diet, Valter Longo, PhD

*Fast Food Genocide, Joel Fuhrman, M.D.

*Eat To Live, Joel Fuhrman, M.D.

*End of Dieting, Joel Fuhrman, M.D.

Disease and Delusion, Dr. Jeffrey Bland

WHOLE, Rethinking The Science of Nutrition, T. Colin Campbell PhD and Howard Jacobson PhD

Glucose Revolution, Jessie Inchauspe

Eat To Beat Disease, William W. Li

The China Study, T. Colin Campbell, PhD and Thomas M. Campbell II, M.D.

*The China Study Solution, Thomas Campbell, M.D.

The Obesity Code, Jason Fung, M.D.

Prescription for Nutritional Healing, Phyllis A Balch, CNC

*Deeply Wholistic, Pip Waller

The Disease Delusion, Dr. Jeffrey S. Bland

The Auto Immune Fix, Tom O'Bryan, DC, CCN, DACBN

Body Into Balance, Maria Noel Groves

What Your Doctor May Not Tell You About Heart Disease, Mark C. Houston, M.D., M.S.

Diet For A New America, John Robbins

Emotional and Mental Resources

These books are a great start to powerfully clearing the path of your personal journey and getting just the kick in the ass you need to become the greater version of yourself. I can attribute so much of my success, happiness, and peacefulness to the study of these incredible resources. I pray they have the same effect for you. Enjoy!

I am a big fan of Mel Robins which is why I've included so many of her books. She is raw and uncensored but really changed my life, along with my mother's and my sister's. I hope you enjoy her as much as we do.

*The Five Second Rule, Mel Robbins

*High Five Habit, Mel Robbins

*Kick Ass With Mel Robbins, Mel Robbins

*Work It Out, Mel Robbins

The Power of One More, Ed Mylett

Just Listen, Mark Goulston

The Magic of Manifesting, Ryuu Shinohara

The Power of Discipline, Daniel Walter

The Mountain is You, Brianna West

*Feel The Fear And Do It Anyway, Susan Jeffers, PhD

Meant For More, Lisa Sasevich

Put Your Ass Where Your Heart Wants To Be, Steven Pressfield

Atomic Habits, James Clear

Mind Set, Carol S. Deweck PhD

The Female Brain, Louann Brizendine M.D.

The Male Brain, Louann Brizendine M.D.

The Buddha and The Badass, Vishen Lakhiani

Allison Armstrong

Last, but not least, Allison Armstrong. I have taken every class Allison has taught and I can say without a doubt she is the authority on understanding men and women. These classes and books helped clear up a lot of mental clutter regarding relationship BS with the men and women in my life including family, friends, romantic partnerships, and work relationships. She is entertaining and seriously impactful.

*Understanding Women, Allison Armstrong

*Understanding Men, Allison Armstrong

*Understanding Partnership, Allison Armstrong

Meditation

Online guided meditations are my personal preference but there are so many options. Here is a list to get you started. You will have to try a few different kinds of meditations and customize what works for you.

YouTube – There are hundreds of guided meditations on YouTube, including Meditations for prayer. Take a look around and try some focused on your specific needs. I do several different ones based on what my needs are for the day.

Headspace - Google Play, Meditation for Beginners

One Commune - www.onecommune.com

CALM - An app you can download and have on your phone or iPAD, this is an excellent resource for affirmations, guided and unguided meditations.

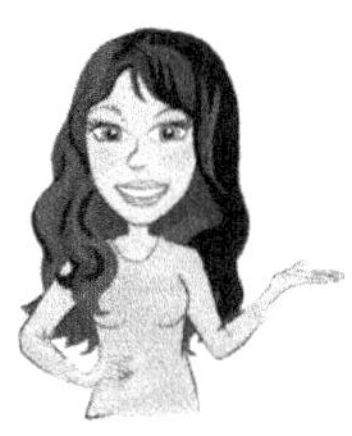

If you feel you need additional support to help you through your journey, as I have mentioned several times, it is an expression of self-love when you recognize an issue might be bigger than you can handle on your own.

Here are some resources right at your fingertips to help get support.

BetterHelp – www.betterhelp.com

Best Online Therapy Services - www.bestonline-therapyservices.com

Top10.com - www.top10.com

Lightfully Behavioral Health - www.lightfully.com

988 Suicide and Crisis Lifeline - www.988lifeline.org

National Institute of Health - www.nimh.nih.gov

Domestic Abuse Hotline – 1-800-799-7233

National domestic violence Hotline – www.thehotline.org

Alcohol Abuse Hotline – 1-844-714-7186

Al-Anon – www.al-anon.org